LIFE REFRAMING IN HYPNOSIS

ABOUT THE AUTHOR

Milton H. Erickson received his MD from the University of Wisconsin. He was President of the American Society of Clinical Hypnosis and a Life Fellow of the American Psychiatric Association and the American Psychopathological Association. Dr Erickson was the founder and editor of the *American Journal of Clinical Hypnosis* and the co-author of *Hypnotic Realities, Hypnotherapy, Experiencing Hypnosis* and *Time Distortion in Hypnosis*. He received the Benjamin Franklin Gold Medal of the International Society of Clinical and Experimental Hypnosis.

ABOUT THE EDITORS

Ernest L. Rossi received his Ph.D from Temple University. He is a Diplomate in Clinical Psychology, a Jungian analyst and a pioneer in psychobiological theory. He is the author of *Dreams and the Growth of Personality* and co-author of *Hypnotic Realities, Hypnotherapy, Experiencing Hypnosis*. He is also editor of *Psychological Perspectives*, a journal of Jungian thought.

Margaret O. Ryan is a graduate in psychology from the University of California. She is a writer, and has edited a number of volumes in the field of psychotherapy and transpersonal psychology.

LIFE REFRAMING IN HYPNOSIS

THE SEMINARS, WORKSHOPS, AND LECTURES OF MILTON H. ERICKSON

VOLUME II

By
Milton H. Erickson

Edited by
Ernest L. Rossi
and
Margaret O. Ryan

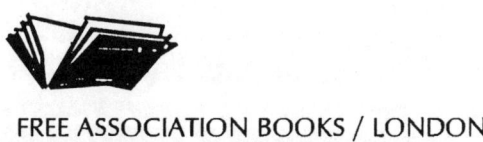

FREE ASSOCIATION BOOKS / LONDON

This edition first published in 1998 by
FREE ASSOCIATION BOOKS
57 Warren Street, London W1P 5PA

Copyright © 1985 by Ernest L. Rossi, Ph.D

All rights reserved. No part of this publication may be reproduced in any manner whatever, including information storage or retrieval, in whole or in part (except for brief quotations in critical articles or reviews), without written permission from the publisher. For information write to Irvington Publishers, Inc., 522, E. 82nd Street, Suite 1, New York, NY 10028, USA.

ISBN 1 85343 406 X

A CIP catalogue record for this book is available from the British Library.

Printed in the EC by J.W. Arrowsmith, Bristol

CONTENTS

Prefatory Notes ... xi

Introduction ... xiii

Part I ... 1
   Utilizing Natural Life Experience for Creative Problem Solving

Part II ... 133
   Reframing Problems into Constructive Activity

Part III ... 189
   New Frames of Reference for Old

Part IV ... 223
   Special States of Awareness and Receptivity

Part V ... 243
   Life Reframing: The Hypnotherapeutic Facilitation of Potentials in a Young Photographer (audio cassette tape)

References ... 301

Bibliography ... 309

Index ... 312

Photos ... 132a
   Milton H. Erickson: A Photographic Portfolio: 1910-1980

DEDICATION

This volume is dedicated to

GREGORY BATESON

and all the workers of the
Mental Research Institute
of Palo Alto, California:
Janet Beavin
Richard Fisch
Jay Haley
Don Jackson
Lynn Segal
Paul Watzlawick
John Weakland

whose development of the heuristic
concepts of the double bind, symptom
prescription, and reframing has
revolutionized our understanding of
the interactional process of change
in psychotherapy

ACKNOWLEDGMENTS

The Editors wish to thank the many individuals who have contributed audio tapes and made valuable suggestions for this volume. Among them:

Seymour Hershman
Herbert Mann
Louis Moore
Marion Moore
Robert Pearson
Irving Secter
Florence Sharp
Kay Thompson
Richard Van Dyck
Jeffrey Zeig

We also wish to acknowledge the help and support of many members from the following societies:

The American Society of Clinical Hypnosis
The Milton H. Erickson Foundation
The Northern California Society of Clinical Hypnosis
The Southern California Society of Clinical Hypnosis

Please note that audio tapes are only available from
Irvington Publishers Inc.,
522 E. 82nd Street, Suite 1, New York, NY 10028, USA

PREFATORY NOTES

Regarding References

Because of the informal nature of the material, the editors decided to use footnotes at the end of the book rather than the standard APA format for referencing. To simplify frequent references to previous Erickson/Rossi volumes, only abbreviated titles are used in the text. Full publication information can be found in the Bibliography.

Regarding the Index

While the editors continue to disavow any effort to systematize Erickson's material in these volumes, we have made a careful effort to catalogue the subject matter in two ways. First we have provided frequent headings which appear in bold face type every page or two to focus attention on the major theme that Erickson is presenting. *These headings are the editors' efforts to catalogue—not Erickson's.* The contents in these headings are then used to select key subject words for the index. *The index is thus the key to the subject matter in these volumes,* and can serve as a reference tool for future scholars who wish to study what Erickson had to say in any particular area.

Regarding the Typesetting

To indicate Erickson's frequent shifts of attention during demonstrations from subjects to audience and back to subjects, all verbatim trance material spoken directly to subjects is in bold face type. His shifts of focus back to the audience are indicated by additional spacing and regular (Roman) type. It should be noted, however, that although addressing the audience, many of Erickson's remarks are being directed to the subjects as forms of indirect suggestions. Lastly, any added commentary by the editors (indented from ongoing text) was written in 1983 without the benefit of prior discussion with Erickson.

INTRODUCTION

This second volume of Milton H. Erickson's seminars, workshops, and lectures is an incredibly rich presentation of his ingenious approaches to hypnosis and psychotherapy. It was during the time period covered by this volume that Erickson wrote some of his most original papers on the *naturalistic* and *utilization* techniques which are considered to be the essence of his approach. It was Erickson's genius to find in the natural patterns of everyday behavior the secrets of each patient's individuality which he then utilized for therapeutic purposes. The stories and anecdotes he tells about his friends, family, colleagues, and patients in this volume provide a delightful tapestry illustrating just how his creative mind went about the process of scientific discovery and hypnotherapeutic innovation.

This volume, therefore, will be most appreciated by students, professionals, and interested readers who are seeking a model that can facilitate their own creative efforts, whatever their special field of endeavor. The psychological insights contained herein have relevance for all who are engaged in expanding the growing edge of human consciousness.

As with the first volume in this series, the presentation of the material is not systematic in the traditional academic sense. Rather we follow along as colleagues while Milton demonstrates in his evocative manner just how he goes about his work. It is this natural path of unsystematic discovery that can be of most value in facilitating the reader's own creative activity.

As the material of this volume was edited for publication, new insights became apparent. The most significant of these was the serendipituous formulation of the now popular concept of *reframing**, which occurred during this period as Milton struggled to tell his audiences just how he went about helping people break out of their learned limitations. In fact, *reframing* can now be seen as a direct consequence of Erickson's naturalistic and utilization approaches. *Therapy, symptom resolution, habit retraining and the reconstruction of personality were effected not by traditional analysis as formulated by Freud, but by the often quixotic process of reframing: reorganizing and reinterpreting the significance and meaning in a person's life experience so that potentials and behavior could be utilized and expressed in a more felicitous manner.* This concept leads us to the view that "psychological problems" are simply unfortunate ways of understanding or *reframing* a situation. Reframing is a way of helping people reorganize their understandings of a situation such that all relevant aspects of it are brought under control.

Certainly science proceeds in this manner: a well-designed experiment is actually a reframing of nature's variables in a way that permits the scientist to systematically control and study them. We could speculate that this is also the essential task of the artist, who helps us reorganize the way we see, hear, feel, and experience the world. Philosophical studies and spiritual practices could probably proceed most effectively in the same manner: by continually reframing our innermost experiences on ever more subtle levels, we have a means of progressively evolving our own human nature.

From a broad historical perspective we now can see the significance of Erickson's contribution to the field of psychotherapy and human development. Sigmund Freud's major contribution was to illustrate how *analysis* and *insight* into the relationship between one's conscious and unconscious processes could be of therapeutic value in freeing a person from neurotic and symptomatic blocks. Freud's early students—Otto Rank,

---

*The term *reframing* was explicated by Paul Watzlawick, John Weakland, and Richard Fisch in their book, *Change: Principles of Problem Formation and Problem Resolution* (New York: W.W. Norton, 1974), for which Erickson wrote a foreword.

Sandor Ferenczi, and Karl Abraham—and the later ego psychologists, such as Karen Horney with her "New Ways of Growth," illustrated how the various symptoms of functional psychopathology were actually aspects of the creative process gone astray via neurotic distortion.

Carl Jung added the concept of an *archetypal collective unconscious* which could be accessed through the methods of *amplification* and *comparative study*. These methods revealed how the personal imagery and ideas of individual patients paralleled the myths and rituals recorded throughout history. His work illustrates how the interaction between the individual and society is an active process of synthesizing new meaning to sustain culture and expand consciousness.

The Gestalt psychologists from Kohler to Fritz Pearls focused on the ability to shift frames of reference and find new orientations and meanings as the essence of creativity in psychotherapy. Humanistic psychologists such as Abraham Maslow and current transpersonal psychologists such as Ken Wilber are broadening this base by integrating our understanding of man on the behavioral, mental, and spiritual levels.

Incredibly rich and valuable as this entire panorama is, there is nonetheless something missing from the point of view of practical psychotherapy. How often have all these insights and meanings helped people understand themselves better while leaving them still unable to change their actual behavior? It is precisely into this breach that Erickson makes his unique contribution: he shows us the actual approaches, methods, and techniques that enable people to utilize their own life experiences and unconsciously learned associations to change behavior, recreate identity, and reframe their lives in new and meaningful ways.

From the first volume of this series we learned how Erickson's personal struggles with sensory-perceptual handicaps and two bouts of poliomyelitis were major motivating factors in the development of his therapeutic approaches. He truly was a living example of the archetype of the wounded physician who learns to heal others only by first learning to heal himself. For those who were fortunate to study with him, that concept was a basic message that always came through on a very personal level: heal thyself, and then teach that healing method to others. In bringing this series of volumes on Erickson's seminars, workshops and lectures to the public, we hope to share this healing with all who can use it personally and help to spread it further.

Ernest Lawrence Rossi
Malibu, 1984

PART I

UTILIZING NATURAL LIFE EXPERIENCE FOR CREATIVE PROBLEM SOLVING*

The Nature of the Unconscious

Utilization of Favorable Experiences in Hypnosis: "You Are My Girl Now"

Everything I say today will be essentially impromptu. I hope from time to time to repeat the important ideas, because if you want to learn, you need to have things repeated.

Now, the first issue I want to discuss is the general attitude that all of you—whether psychologists, dentists, or physicians—ought to have in regard to the utilization of hypnosis and its significance to the individual patient. In hypnosis one is employing primarily the unconscious or the subconscious mind. I will probably use those terms interchangeably throughout this lecture. A great deal has been written on the subject of the unconscious, the subconscious, and the preconscious, but the idea I wish to impress upon you is this: that *the unconscious mind is that part of the mind that deals primarily with symbolic thinking in which there is no need for external reality orientation but in which there is the capacity for such orientation.* Thus, a person can think about a glass of water with his unconscious mind. He can visualize it very, very clearly without the concrete prop of the glass of water. Just the thought, the idea,

---

*Presentation given in San Diego, California in February of 1958.

the memory, the understanding of a glass of water is sufficient for the unconscious mind.

Now, the next point that I want to make is this: *The unconscious mind is the storehouse for all personality experiences, personality learnings, and personality attitudes.* We are all influenced by our total backgrounds. In the past, however, too much emphasis has been placed upon the traumatic aspects of everyday living. Too much emphasis has been focused on the possibilities for traumatizing people, on the possibilities for being affected unfavorably by this sort of experience or that sort of experience. Too little attention has been given to the question of the effect of something favorable upon a person's life—the effect of something very, very pleasing to the person. Just as a horribly traumatic experience can condition a person with tremendous force and rigidity, so can a pleasant experience.

I will give you an example from my own personal background. Some 72 years ago—you wonder how my personal background got into this!—a 16-year-old boy was riding in an ox cart on his way to a foster home. The ox cart stopped at a farm. While the driver went into the farmhouse this 16-year-old boy, who had run away from his brother's home in Chicago, looked all around at the Wisconsin farmlands. A young girl peeped out from behind a maple tree. The 16-year-old boy said, "Whose girl are you?" The girl replied very coyly (she was 13), "I'm my daddy's girl." The 16-year-old boy promptly announced: "You are my girl now."

Seven years later my father married the girl from behind the maple tree. But it had all been settled right then and there. They have been happily married for 65 years. That one little statement which my mother recorded in her diary preserves the incident very, very nicely and shows the tremendous and lasting influence any favorable event from the past can have.

When you are using hypnosis with patients, realize that the fashion in which you appeal to the unconscious mind establishes a foundation for your patients' future thinking and feeling—about hypnosis, about dentistry, about medicine, about their bodies, about how they react to physical and mental distress. With this understanding, you can then appreciate the tremendous need for using hypnosis in a way that emphasizes the pleasurable things of life for your patients. Now I stress this because you need to teach your patients not to be too concerned about fear and anxiety. But before I take up that issue I want to mention one other consideration in the use of hypnosis.

Utilizing a "Reserve Bank" of Life Experiences

Extrapolating Posthypnotic Suggestion to Cover All Future Contingencies of Menstrual Distress

Whether you are pulling a tooth, lancing a carbuncle, or whatever it happens to be—no matter how simple or how complicated—you ought to keep the following in mind. Your patient is one person today, quite another person tomorrow, and still another person next week, next month, next year. Five years from now, ten and twenty years from now, he is yet another person. We all have a certain general background, that is true, but we are different persons each day that we live.

I am going to illustrate this point with a clear example. A young woman thirty years of age came to see me. Her complaint was, "I have painful menstruation. I am laid up in bed for three days every month, and I am really thoroughly sick." She told me who her doctor was, and I knew how competent a doctor he was, and I also knew his attitude toward plain and simple neurotic attitudes. I questioned my patient extensively. My feeling was that her three days of disability had profound, psychosomatic origins.

I asked her what she wanted me to do for her, and she replied: "I am going to menstruate in about two weeks, and I don't want to be in bed for three days of vomiting, headaches, and feeling miserable all over. I want you to make sure that I do not have that menstrual difficulty."

"Yes," I said, "but you menstruate about every twenty-eight days, and twenty-eight days from two weeks from now you will have another menstrual period."

She looked at me rather sharply and said, "We are just talking about my next period. That's all."

Now I wondered what was going on in my patient's mind. I reminded her again that menstruation was a thing that occurred every month, this year and next year, too—in fact, five years from now as well. She asked me to tend to the question as she had presented it; that is, to deal only with her next menstrual period. So I gave her suggestions only relating to her next period. And she had a perfectly casual period; no particular discomfort, no pain, no cramps, no loss of time from her job.

I didn't see her for another six weeks. Then she came in and said, "That period you treated me for was a perfectly delightful menstrual period. My next one was on time, but I was in bed for three whole days, horribly ill. In fact, I think I caught up on all the sickness I missed the period you treated me for."

"Yes," I said, "I rather expected that to happen. Why didn't you let me give you suggestions for future periods?"

"I wanted to find out for myself," she answered.

She was correct in that attitude. But now she was willing to allow me to suggest that she could have relief and freedom from all menstrual difficulties: from premenstrual and postmenstrual difficulties for her next period, and for all subsequent menstrual periods this year, next year, for five years, for ten years, until menopause arrived.

She interrupted me to say, "But I still have the right to have menstrual distress."

"Yes, that is right, you do."

This patient was exceedingly understanding, and therefore I continued: "Any time you want to have menstrual pain and distress, simply remember that it is your period, it is your menstruation. Remember that it is your menstrual pain, your menstrual cramps, your menstrual distress. Any time you wish to have difficulty, it is your privilege to do so; and I want you to bear that squarely in mind."

The patient was very, very pleased that I, in doing therapy

with her, had given her *the privilege of keeping available a sort of reserve in her bank of life experiences*—a reserve of menstrual distress to be used any time she wanted to use it. She didn't know when or why she might want to use it in the future, but it was important to know that she could if she wanted or needed to.

Posthypnotic Suggestion for Future Life Changes

Next I presented for her understanding an idea she had not considered. Actually it is an idea which most doctors and dentists don't consider in their approach to patients. Whether the problem is menstrual pain, denture pain, or whatever: [patients and their life circumstances will change over time].

I explained: "You may get married some time. You may get pregnant. You may not get married. You may have a severe attack of pneumonia that will interfere with your period, and so you will have an interruption of your menstrual cycle. Bear in mind that everything I have said about this matter of therapy for your regular menstruation does not extend just up to a skipped period or to a time of no periods, but it extends beyond. If you get married and get pregnant, there will be a total interruption of your menstrual cycle. You will be a different person after you get married, get pregnant, have the baby, nurse the baby. You will be totally different physiologically, psychologically, and somatically. When your menstruation resumes after your baby is born you need to understand that everything I have said about menstruation today, here in the office, applies to you as the mother of a child; applies to you as a person who has recovered from a severe bout with pneumonia; applies to you as a person who has experienced anything that interferes with the menstrual period. In other words, no interruption of your menstrual period can terminate the effectiveness of this therapy." She thoroughly understood me!

About six months later she was working for a physician who was known to pay minimal salaries while working his office help very, very hard. The physician's partner went on a vacation and there was a sudden influx of patients resulting in a thoroughly chaotic office. My patient looked the matter over. She knew how useless it would be to ask for a pay raise, so right in the middle of that influx of patients—when the doctor was rushed and overworked—she had a period. And she had a period with all of the former distress and pain and agony, but she bravely continued to work; and she dragged herself around the office so courageously!

The physician who had treated her previously for menstrual difficulties was in the same building and he told her employer that that girl really ought to go to bed. Her employer thought over the situation, and he decided he had better give her a twenty-five—no, better make that fifty—dollar raise. She knew what she was doing!

A year or so later she got married. She was so eager to have a baby that she developed a false pregnancy resulting in a two-month interruption of her cycle. When her period resumed, it was with the former distress and pain until she suddenly recalled in her unconscious mind that I had extended the therapy to cover any and all interruptions.

Posthypnotic Suggestions in Dentistry

Comfortable Denture-Wear Now and in the Future

The same idea applies in the field of dentistry. You ought to be willing to teach your patient to wear those dentures today, next week, next year. And whenever he changes dentures, do you want him to go through a struggling period of re-learning how? You pull a tooth or two. Do you want to re-teach that same patient this matter of a balanced bite? Do you want to re-teach him the proper way to accommodate himself to eating when he's got a missing tooth or two? You need to recognize that all patients change.

Now and then I get patients who come to me to be hypnotized so that they can readjust to their new set of dentures. They were used to their old ones, but there have been some changes in their mouths and so they have to get new sets of dentures. At the present time, I can refer them to the dentists in the Arizona Society of Clinical Hypnosis. But I want you to understand that *whenever you deal with patients, you deal with them not only in terms of the immediate present but also in terms of future perspectives and possibilities.*

Approaches to Pain and Anxiety

Acknowledging the Truth of Distress; Shifting the Focus of Attention; Reframing Distress: Robert's "Right" to As Many Stitches as Possible!

Let's discuss this matter of alleviating fear and anxiety. The direct frontal attack is the most common method of approaching a patient. We all have learned from childhood onward to tell the injured or sick person: "It doesn't hurt," or "You'll feel better shortly." Our tendency is to contradict the reality of the patient's suffering: "You don't need to be afraid ... I'm not going to hurt you ... This Novocain will really fix you up ... You won't notice this local anesthetic much," and so on. But all of these statements are absolutely contrary to the personal experience of the patient.

I am going to illustrate this point by using my son Robert's experience. Robert was about three years old at the time. He fell down the back steps and split his lower lip horribly, knocking an upper tooth up into the maxilla. There he lay shouting to high heaven, announcing to the entire neighborhood his pain and distress and fright. He had good lungs! Mrs. Erickson and I went out to see what all the hubbub was. By this time Robert was really yelling, so what sense would it make to tell him to stop crying? He would know immediately that I just didn't understand. Would it make any sense for me to tell him it didn't hurt, when with every fiber of his being he knew that it hurt? It was *his* jaw, *his* lip, *his* face, *his* mouth that were hurting him, and he knew it!

Now how could I communicate with that little 3-year-old boy? There was only one way—the same way that I would communicate with a grown-up person. I told Robert, "It hurts just awful, just terrible, doesn't it?" He knew I was talking sense. He knew from his own experience that it was hurting awfully, it was hurting terribly; and he now knew that I was an intelligent observer and so he could listen to me. Then very promptly I added, "And it is continuing to hurt." Another intelligent remark on my part with which he could agree.

In your approach to patients with fear, anxiety, and pain you need to have them recognize that you agree with them and that they can agree with you. When I told Robert that his injury was continuing to hurt I was expressing a fear—I was expressing a knowledge—that he and I possessed in common and upon which we thoroughly agreed. Next I said the obvious thing, "And you wish it would stop hurting." Naturally he would wish for it to stop hurting! He knew that I understood that he wished it would stop hurting. Having raised that issue I could add, "And maybe it will stop in a little while, or in a minute or two." I had acknowledged what he was wishing for and I was suggesting that he would have his wish "in a little while." I did not say "right away." I put it in a time framework he could believe—"in a little while." All of us have learned that "in a little while" this will happen, that will happen. It is in accord with our total understanding of things—with out total lifetime of learnings—that "in a little while" such and such will happen. Then you can redefine that little while to a minute or two. How long is a minute or two? Everyone knows that for a little child a minute or two can be immediate or hours long, depending upon the subjective experience. Robert knew I was talking sense. Maybe it would stop hurting, and all his past experience had taught him that sometimes pain did stop—in fact that all pain did stop—after a while.

Having presented those ideas to Robert my next task was to present yet another set of ideas. You see, whether you are working with experimental subjects in the psychology lab, with dental patients, with obstetrical patients, or with psychiatric patients, you need to present ideas in such a way that they can respond to those ideas in such a total fashion that they are not responding to other alien and undesirable ideas. Since I had just presented to Robert the idea that maybe it would stop hurting in a little while, or in a minute or two, I now presented another idea. I looked at the sidewalk and asked Mrs. Erickson if the blood on it was good, strong, red blood. She looked at the sidewalk, and she looked at the blood stains. Now this was an earnest question; this was a serious question. Never mind what I as a physician know about blood. Robert was just three years old, and it was his blood that was under discussion. Therefore I wanted to know if his blood was good, strong, red blood. I looked at it, Mrs. Erickson looked at it, and Mrs. Erickson said she thought it was fine blood. I looked from this patch of blood here over to that patch of blood there, and then I compared which was the redder. But, of course, you can't tell how really red the blood is because the sidewalk is the wrong color. So I told Mrs. Erickson to pick up Robert and take him into the bathroom where we would let him bleed into the white sink in the bathroom. Then we would be able to see if the blood was good, strong, red blood.

Now when you are three years old you want good, strong, red blood. There is nothing finer, as any red-blooded American knows! So now Robert was interested in being taken into the bathroom. I rinsed out the sink, ran the water, and let him drip into the sink. I pointed out that with that running of water into his blood it made a nice pink color. But maybe I'd better turn off the faucet and just look at the red blood itself. We both looked and we both agreed that it was good, strong, red blood, and I poured some water over his head to thin it out again and see if it was a perfectly good pink. It was a perfectly good pink. So Robert got his face washed, and I was able to stop the flow of blood. Then I broke some awfully bad news to Robert, but I broke that news in the way you really ought to approach patients. I told Robert that I didn't think his lip was cut enough to require as many stitches as Betty Alice, his sister, bragged about owning. And I didn't think he could have as many stitches as his brother Alan bragged about owning, but I did want him to see to it that he counted those stitches and that the surgeon put in as many stitches as possible. I didn't tell him *not* to feel pain. Instead I told him to see to it that stitches were put in and to carefully count those stitches as they were being put in. So it became not a task in which he avoided feeling pain; it became a task in which he insisted on his right to as many stitches as possible. I pointed out that I was even afraid he wouldn't get as many stitches as he could count. To his profound disgust he only got seven stitches! He had wanted ten but only got seven; and Allan had gotten over thirty stitches, and Betty Alice had gotten over fifty-two; and the surgeon looked at that little 3-year-old who was protesting his insufficient stitching!

In this matter of fear, anxiety, pain, and distress, you never try to falsify the situation in a direct way. Sneak around from behind to falsify or alter the actuality by giving your patient some other idea to consider and respond to. But never deny the validity, the genuineness, of a patient's experience. Recognize that he does have pain, he does have fear, he does have anxiety; and it is only right, it is only just, that you admit to him that you know those facts. *You never ask the patient to falsify his own understanding; instead you give him other understandings that nullify, that contradict, that absorb and hold his focus, so that he cannot give all his attention to what is distressing him.*

> Eds: These "other understandings" are actually what we would now call "new frames of reference." The hypnotherapist helps the patient *reframe* the distressful experience so that it is nullified, restructured, or otherwise shifted out of the focus of attention.[1]

Facilitating the Freedom to Experience

Time Binds in Dentistry: A Slap in the Face

I am going to mention another example. I know of three dentists—a California dentist, an Eastern dentist, and a Midwestern dentist—who all use the same approach. They each explained to me that when you get a child in the office who is afraid of the dentist you do the following. When the child starts yelling and screaming, you clamp a towel over his mouth, hold him rigidly, and explain to him as he chokes and sputters in his fear and terror that you will have to continue doing so until he quiets down and cooperates. All three of those dentists told me that after one such experience the child becomes very, very cooperative and very, very friendly and agreeable—even to the point of wanting to come back. I don't blame the child for being friendly; I don't blame the child for wanting to come back: he has learned that a dentist approaches a child with force, and one such experience with one such dentist is enough! Why go through it again! He had better just come back to this one. He had better be friendly, he had better be cooperative, or he will get that towel over his face again. He had better put up with anything; he had better be friendly and cheerful and cooperative, against a background of terror.

So I disagree with that approach to the child (or adult) who is fearful, tense, screaming, or anything else. I can think of the 21-year-old woman who walked into the dental office of a friend of mine and said, "I want to see your office; I want to see where you have your office desk; I don't want to see you; I want to see where you've got your dental chair."

My friend said, "All right, but can you tell me why?"

"The last time I went to the dentist," she said, "was when I was a little girl. That dentist slapped my face until I stopped crying, and now I need some dental care, and I am really scared. I am awfully scared, and I need dental care. I would like to have you look in my mouth and tell me how much I need, but please don't slap my face."

My dentist-friend sat down behind his desk and said: "Suppose you lean back in your chair and I'll lean back in mine. You are really afraid of me, aren't you? But aren't you glad that there is this distance between us? And you really like to hang onto the arms of that chair, because you are so scared."

He let that girl discover exactly how scared she was, and exactly how comforting it was that she was far away from him on the other side of a very wide desk. He brought that fear and that anxiety out into the open where the girl couldn't possibly conceal or falsify any of her subjective responses. The girl realized that the dentist wasn't going to falsify the situation; that he, in fact, was going to encourage her sympathetically to feel her fear, and to feel it in his presence. He wasn't going to tell her, "Nonsense, you don't need to be afraid of me." *Once the patient had the freedom to feel afraid, she also had the freedom to feel comfortable and to develop a sense of trust.*

Next my dental-friend asked her: *"When do you think you would like to have your appointment? Don't suggest too early an appointment, but postpone it just as long as you wish."*

> Eds: This is a basic time bind: the patient is given a choice about *when* she will have an appointment—but when she makes that choice she thereby binds herself into accepting an appointment. Notice the subtlety of the two essential characteristics of the time bind: (1) she is given free choice, but (2) when exercising her free choice she *binds herself.* Her own free choice (which has a positive feeling tone) determines and commits her behavior. The dentist does not bind her; he merely gives her an opportunity—a choice—to bind herself. Thus we can understand how binds and double binds are actually new forms of human interaction that do not depend upon power and control in the traditional sense. Binds and double binds offer individuals the means of making creative choices to modify their own behavior in a manner that they themselves find desirable. Binds and double binds offer patients an opportunity to overcome their own resistances, unfortunate life experiences, and/or complexes. *Binds and double binds in these therapeutic circumstances are not a means of controlling or manipulating patients against their wills.* If this patient did not want to experience dentistry she would have no trouble at all in resisting the time bind that was offered.[2]

This gave the girl the freedom to delay it, and so she said, "Would it be all right if I put it off until tomorrow?"

"Let's make it *late* tomorrow," he responded, thus postponing it even more. But, you know, *late* tomorrow is really pretty soon. By emphasizing *late* tomorrow he was accommodating her need to put it off into the future—tomorrow. She was so afraid it would be today, and then he emphasized that *lateness* of tomorrow. He climbed on board her own particular bandwagon; he took her understandings of delay and emphasized them.

Next he asked her: "At your first appointment late tomorrow, do you want me just to look in your mouth and see what is there, or do you want me to examine the left lower side?" He was cutting it up—making it a small issue.

"Well," the patient answered, "you could look at all of the left side—I suppose you could look at all of it and examine all of it."

And he agreed that he would examine the lower left side, and if there were time enough he would examine whatever more was possible in that length of time. Remember, the girl hadn't set foot inside a dentist's office since the age of eight. She was terrified.

The girl came in the next day for her appointment and said, "I want you to go into the regular office—not the office where the dental chair is."

So he went in and sat down on the far side of the desk, and she said, "Can we sit here for a while?"

"Oh, yes," he said, "a minute or two, or even five minutes, six or seven. It really doesn't make any difference how long we sit here."

Notice that while he had specified a top limit of seven minutes, he had also said, "It really doesn't make any difference how long we sit here." Thus he established both a minimal and maximal time limit [but within the comforting framework that "it really doesn't make any difference how long we sit here"]. Whenever you use hypnosis, understand what you say, and specify limits: a maximum of seven minutes, a minimum of—it doesn't make any difference.

> Eds: This *time binding choice* apparently satisfies both sides of the patient's ambivalence and her need for control: her wish to delay the examination as long as possible is satisfied by "It really doesn't make any difference how

long we sit here"; her wish to have the examination is satisfied by specifying the time limits within which it will be done—"a minute or two, or even five minutes, six or seven." Giving the patient all these time choices also provides her with some control in an anxiety-provoking situation where she formerly had none.

Fixating Attention with Light and Touch

Indirect Hypnotic Induction via Touch and Distraction in Dentistry

Within a minute's time she said, "Take me by the hand and lead me in. I'll sit down in that dental chair."

So my dentist-friend took her in, and as he did so he remarked on the mirror and the light. He stressed that mirror and that light. And she sat there. He explained how the lighting involved a rather complex process of arrangement in order to produce a light that created no shadows so that it would shine on this side of the mouth, on that side of the mouth; so that the reflected light would cover the lower part of the mouth, the upper part of the mouth, the right and the left. Now the girl consciously thought that he was talking about the light, but her unconscious knew that he was really talking about the lower part of her mouth, the upper part of her mouth, the right and the left. And as the girl continued to hold onto the dentist's hand, he, of course, was employing that touch technique of inducing a trance. He was fixating the girl's attention on the light; he was fixating the girl's attention on her wrist; he was limiting and focusing her attention onto herself and her growing feeling of comfort. He wasn't forcing her. He just gave her other things to respond to, with the result that he was able to relax one arm and put it on the arm of the chair; he was able to relax the other arm and put it there; to relax her neck by putting her head back; to relax her shoulders; and to relax her neck even further by opening her mouth and relaxing the platysma muscle. And it sounded so good to the girl—just relaxing that platysma muscle.

The dentist made no effort to reassure her. But he did make an effort to present to her the distance between her chair and his chair; the light that she could look at, the mirror that she could look at; the relaxation of one arm and then the other arm that she could enjoy; the relaxation of the back of her neck, the front of her neck; the alleviation of her fear and anxiety by the offer to examine the lower left part of her mouth, and whatever else could be examined in the time at his disposal and at her disposal.

After the dentist examined her mouth—he did a very complete examination—he told the girl that she didn't have a sound tooth in her head. All of her teeth were frightfully corroded; after all, she had not brushed her teeth since that one horrible slapping she'd received as a little girl in that dental office. She had neglected her teeth horribly, and every tooth was horribly decayed. He told her that she would have to have an extraction and that she would undoubtedly need to have an anesthesia. He explained that there were several types of anesthesia, all the way from hypnosis to Novocain, and he named all the possible anesthetic agents. He didn't try to tell her that she was in a decidedly good, light-to-medium trance at the time, because he had put her in the trance without her awareness. He had used gentleness and a presentation of ideas to occupy her attention.

Presenting Ideas

Indirect Ideodynamic Focusing to Achieve Dental Goals

I am enlarging upon this dental situation because the same principle applies to any psychological situation that confronts the professional. It applies clinically; and it also applies experimentally in the psychologist's laboratory in the carrying out of physiological experiments. The principle is simply that of presenting ideas to secure and enlist the wholehearted cooperation of whomever you are working with.

The dental patient I just described certainly enjoyed the entire situation, yet at no time did the dentist tell her she need not be afraid; at no time did he tell her she need not feel a thing. He explained how he could use this anesthetic agent, that anesthetic agent; he could tell her the formula of this and the formula of that: "This anesthetic requires a syringe and needle to administer, but that anesthetic can be dropped onto the skin to produce a numbness. And with hypnosis, you also can produce a numbness on the surface of the skin, but actually, an anesthesia of the entire arm is produced so that you forget entirely where your arm is." And then he began talking about her jaw, while she proceeded to forget about where her arm was.

Too often in the professional use of hypnosis there is that direct driving toward a specific goal, when actually it is more effective to just mention your goal. You do not keep reminding the patient, "I want you to have an anesthesia in your right hand, which has four fingers and one thumb on it and is attached to the wrist"! You merely mention that it is perfectly possible to get an anesthesia in the hand, and then you discuss anesthesia from other points of view: glove anesthesia, chemoanesthesia, hypnotic anesthesia. You are mentioning anesthesia, and how many times do you have to say, "anesthesia of the hand"? You say it once, and then you drive home on the general subject of anesthesia. The patient's unconscious mind understands and carries out what you are indirectly driving at.

> Eds: This is the principle of *indirect ideodynamic focusing*.[3] A simple discussion of the many varieties of anesthesia will automatically and indirectly stimulate the unconscious to explore its various psychophysiological mechanisms for evoking anesthesia. The *idea* of anesthesia automatically evokes the *psychophysiological responses* of anesthesia. These psychophysiological responses are either inhibited in everyday life, or simply pass unnoticed by us. In the hypnotic situation, "suggestion" simply permits these inherent "background" psychophysiological responses to come to the "forefront" of conscious experience. This is the essence of the naturalistic approach: we arrange circumstances so that the natural, inherent responses of the body-mind are utilized for therapeutic pur-

poses. Hypnotic suggestion does not add or impose anything on the subject: *suggestion merely arranges circumstances and choices so that natural mental mechanisms (that are usually processed in an unconscious manner) are made available for creative and therapeutic purposes.*

A Lifetime of Comfortable Dentures

Questions and Startling Ideas for Facilitating New Attitudes

Our dental patient went back to the dental office to get her upper and lower dentures. And even before the dentist had prepared those dentures for her mouth, he was discussing with her this question of adjusting to her false teeth.

"How long do you think it will take you to learn to wear your dentures? You know, you are in college now; and of course, you are going to wear your dentures on dates, and a pretty girl like you is bound to do some necking. The question that is going to intrigue you fully is, how does it feel for a boy to kiss a girl who wears an upper and a lower plate? How does it feel for a boy to kiss a girl with store-bought teeth? And the answer is rather simple. The boy is going to kiss that girl on her lips."

Now that was a startling idea to her and she then realized that she didn't have to worry too much about her store-bought teeth. Notice, too, how willing that dentist was to use the phrase, *store-bought teeth*. He gave the vulnerable subject the most hideous name possible, but he talked about it so sweetly, so gently, and so pleasingly that there was no opportunity for her to attach an unlovely, personal significance to the phrase. [At the same time, he was discharging whatever fear and resistance she was feeling about her store-bought teeth by "calling them for what they were."][4]

When I next saw her she could talk to me about her store-bought teeth, and she could do so with a pleasant smile and a great deal of pride in the fact that none of the boys who had kissed her had realized that she wore store-bought teeth. Why should they? So she recognized that she had finished a year of college quite successfully, which proved to her that her teeth would not interfere. She would enroll the next year with dentures, and the following year, and the following year. And eventually she would get married, and her false teeth would go with her, and she really had nothing to worry about. And she could even get sick and have to go to the hospital where her teeth would be taken out of her mouth. And as she grew older the taste of foods would change: she could enjoy using those false teeth even when she got beyond that stage of eating as a 21-year-old and began eating as a 40-year-old, with a different set of food values and tastes. In short, she was given a rather comprehensive summary of the possible experiences with those false teeth, as she would encounter the different events to come in her life. This allowed her to acquire her false teeth as something that she would have with her and that she could enjoy, despite changes in her life.

Believing in Hypnosis

Depotentiating Fear of Hypnosis via Acceptance and Positive Expectancy

One always approaches this matter of fear and anxiety directly, and without trying to contradict it. There is no sense in trying to tell a person that he is not afraid; no sense in telling him he is not anxious, he is not fearful—because he is. He knows it, he understands it, and he believes it. All you achieve by disputing your patient's obvious reality is the arousal of his disbelief and distrust—and above all, you want your patient to believe you.

When patients come to you for the first time, they do not necessarily understand or believe in hypnosis. The dental patient was a different matter. Her sister had been a patient of mine and had spoken about hypnosis, so she was prepared. But when patients come to you who do not believe in hypnosis, I don't think you ought to announce, "Well, I do!" Do not brag about your confidence in hypnosis. Explain instead, "I really expect you not to believe fully in hypnosis because you personally haven't had the experience yet."

> Eds: This simple statement is a masterpiece of indirect suggestion. It contains at least three indirect suggestions: it is a compound sentence with truisms leading to a yes set; it contains the negative; it contains a timebinding implication in the use of *yet,* etc.[5]

Why should they believe fully in hypnosis when they haven't had the experience yet? What you are telling them is that they are *going* to have the experience; that you really *expect* them to have the experience; and that then they *can believe* in the reality of hypnosis. This is your first, genuine communication to patients. The communication is such that it acknowledges their disbelief in hypnosis and at the same time justifies their expectation that you will use hypnosis to their benefit.

Overcoming Fear

Juxtaposing Negative with Positive Indirect Suggestions to Facilitate Speed of Learning

It is much better for you to announce all the negative issues clearly and openly: "I don't know how quickly you can learn, but then we all have different learning speeds." What are you doing with that statement? You don't know how quickly the individual can learn, but you do know that we all have different learning speeds. You are contrasting a positive statement with a negative statement.

"Some of us learn to type rapidly but to take shorthand very slowly; to drive a car very quickly but to play golf very slowly. We all have different learning speeds, and we differ in our learning speeds for different kinds of learnings." Again, what are you doing with these statements? You are raising the question of a rate of learning, but you used the word *speed*. You haven't said we have different degrees of *slowness* in learning; you've said we have different degrees of *speed* in learning, and so you have suggested a rapidity.

Another: "I do not know how rapidly *you can get over your fear,* but there is no need of rushing too fast." You are emphasizing the fact that there is fear—you may not know how *fast* they can get over it, but there is no sense in *rushing* it—and you are stressing that they are going to get over that fear. They can take all the time in the world, but you still have said *speed,* you still have said *rushing,* and both in relation to the fear.

The same idea applies to anxiety and to disbelief. Disbelief in hypnosis is so often a cover-up for anxiety, a cover-up for fear, a cover-up for a sense of insecurity and uncertainty about the therapeutic situations in which patients find themselves.

> Eds: "I do not know how rapidly *you can get over your fear,* but there is no need of rushing too fast" is another sentence that bristles with several indirect forms of suggestion. *Not knowing* evokes an inner search in the patient; the use of the *negative* in "*no* need of rushing too fast" implies the reverse suggestion, which is interspersed as "you can get over your fear."[5]

Thumbsucking

Hypnotic Suggestion as the Presentation of Response-Evoking Ideas; Nontraumatic Basis of Many Habitual Responses

The next topic I want to discuss is the correction of habits. One ought to approach any teaching situation with patients in essentially the same fashion. Whether the purpose is for an operation, or for the correction of a habit, or for the induction of a hypnotic trance, *your task is to present ideas to patients in such a fashion that they can respond to them.*

Consider thumbsucking. Now, this audience is about half physicians and half dentists; and since I am a physician, since I am a psychiatrist, I feel free to express my opinion on the subject of dentists correcting psychological habits. I think that the vast majority of habits developed by people tend to be habits based on habitual patterns of response, and so they are not necessarily symptomatic of deep traumatic experiences. The thumbsucking starts as a little experimental investigation of the body by the child, and the child finds that he can entertain himself, and so he does it. And the grown-up gets into the habit of fiddling with his pencil as he sits and listens to somebody talk. And I can sit and listen to somebody talk as I fiddle with a pencil, and it is not because I've had a traumatic experience of some sort that compels me to do this, but because I can do it. And I don't have to use a pencil—I can use a pen; when I smoke I can use a cigarette; I can use matches.

Accepting and Utilizing Behavior

Implication Facilitating Responsiveness to Suggestion: Dental and Obstetrical Examples

[At this point there is apparently a question from the audience, which was lost in the recording.]

That is a point I have already mentioned: *the acceptance and utilization of whatever your patient brings to you by way of behavior.*

Let's use the dental setting again. Your patient walks into your dental office, sits down utterly tense, and proceeds to grip the arms of the chair in an utterly tense way. You can plainly see that he is tense, and that both of his hands are gripping the chair. For you to counteract that by asking him to relax his hands is literally an assault upon him. He is tense and he is gripping, and your attitude should be more like the following:

"The way you are gripping that chair actually demonstrates to me that you have a remarkably good grip in that hand. Now, do you mind squeezing a little bit tighter, because I would like to see the muscle play."

You ask the patient to grip the arm of the chair a little bit tighter because you want to see the muscle play. You are asking him to grip that chair, but now it is in response to your request. Therefore, *you have made his tension—his muscle gripping—a part of his responsive behavior to you, and that is what you want. You want everything in the patient's total dental situation to be responsive to you.*

Let's take an obstetrical example. Your OB patient is up on the table in the stirrups, and she starts tightening her thighs. What are you going to do? You really ought to ask her to grip onto the hand-holds and to tighten that little finger just a little bit more. Why do you want the little finger tightened a little bit more? You want that little finger tightened a little bit more on the hand-holds because if she grips tighter with that little finger then by *implication* she is allowing you to suggest the forefinger; she is allowing you to suggest contraction of the biceps; she is allowing you to suggest a movement of any part of her body, including her thighs. And you have pinpointed it all in a nice way by simply asking for control of the little finger. You can approve of gripping with the little finger, and then you can approve of relaxation of the little finger. Then you can suggest the shifting of the position of the entire hand, which, when she complies, will give *you implicit control over all of her muscular behavior.*

Never fight, reject, or try to contradict whatever behavior the patient brings into the office. Instead, you look at it, you examine it, and you wonder how you use it, then you figure out specific ways. With the obstetrical patient you point out that muscle tension in the hand, the arm, and the forearm will be very desirable, while relaxation of the face will also be desirable. But that *implies* muscle tension here, relaxation there; and that is what you want, because she is going to have muscle tension in certain parts of her body.

You also want relaxation in the dental patient, but you want enough muscle tension so that he can lean forward and spit properly into the bowl. You do want some muscle tension. You do not want complete relaxation. *You want control in goal directed behavior for your patient*—no matter what kind of patient you are dealing with.

Overcoming Blocks to Re-entering Trance

Questions for the Revival of Original Trance Situation

Next I want to discuss the approach one takes to the difficult problem of induction of patients you or another doctor have had in a trance previously. There is the patient you have had in a trance before who now comes into your office and says, "Doctor, I don't know what has happened, but for some no-good reason I feel that I can't go into a trance."

Or, there is the patient who says: "I used to go to Doctor So-and-So, but he has moved to another state, and he gave me posthypnotic suggestions so that I cannot go into a trance for anybody else. I would like to have you use hypnosis, but I have been to various other doctors and none of them could hypnotize me. I've just got to write that doctor who left the state—but I don't know his address—to get his permission to go into a trance."

Another variation on this situation is, "I used to be able to go into a deep trance, but I can only go into a light trance now."

In other words, from time to time you will encounter patients who suddenly, for no known reason, simply cannot go into a trance again. What are you going to do? Recently at a seminar I conducted one of the seminarians stated: "I used to go into deep trances, but I have lost the ability. I haven't been able to go into a trance for several years, and I wonder if you can teach me how to go into a trance again. I have tried it repeatedly over the years. I'm always a total failure."

I told the seminarian that I would like to ask him a few questions about his situation: "When was the last time you can remember being in a trance? Where were you sitting at the time? Can you remember if you were sitting in an upholstered chair? Was it upholstered in cloth or leather? By any chance, were you in a doctor's office? Was it a physician's or a dentist's office? Can you remember if the chair you were in faced east or west or north or south? Can you recall just what your eyes were fixed on? Were you sitting up?"

Well, the patient was sitting up in a red leather chair, and he was facing a wall where there was a built-in bookcase. The doctor sat slightly to the left of him, talking to him softly. And he said how he had gone into a deep trance, and I kept on asking those seemingly nonsensical questions—those little details: Could he tell me the title of one of the books in the bookcase? How many shelves did it have? Possibly how wide were the bookcases? And were there pictures on the wall?

As the seminarian answered all my questions, as he recalled those little details, item-by-item, he went into a profound trance—a trance that he was reviving out of the past and transferring into a present trance in rapport with me. That is why I asked him all of those questions. I knew that as surely as he started answering those questions he would reawaken all of his trance feelings from the past—he would literally revive the original trance situation—and thus he would go into a trance. As soon as he was deep enough in the trance I told him that any time in the future he wanted to go into a trance he could do so, and that he could fully enjoy going into that trance. I slowly and gently aroused him without telling him that he had just been in a trance. (The other seminarians in the room had seen that he was in a profound trance, but he, himself, did not know it.) Next I asked him if he really thought he couldn't go into a trance. He answered: "I will come up there and talk to you. I have changed my mind. I think I can go into a trance."

Your willingness to consider your patient in terms of his past experience will enable you to circumvent a lot of these kinds of difficulties.

The Case of Dr. L

Time Distortion Delimiting the Organic, Psychological, and Personality Components of Cancer Pain: Facilitating Neuro-Psychophysiological Responses

What is the value of hypnosis in the treatment of organic lesions? I can give you an example of fairly recent origin by way of an answer.

Perhaps some of you dentists in the audience remember Dr. John L of Phoenix, Arizona. He was an old, old-timer who had several dozen patents on the various dental instruments. He died recently of cancer of the prostate. Before his death he suffered from a generalized carcinomatosis which advanced very rapidly and produced a tremendous amount of pain. Some of you also may remember Dr. Dave Harren at Wayne University College of Dentistry. Dave Harren suggested that I be called in to hypnotize Dr. L.

Now, there was nothing that I, as a psychiatrist, could do about the carcinomatosis—about the metastases—all through the patient's body. Dr. L was dying, he had but a couple of weeks to live, and neither morphine nor Demerol touched his pain. Furthermore, Dr. L didn't like the idea of being so thoroughly narcoticized that he couldn't spend the last two weeks, conscious, with his family. I saw that he had a tremendous motivation to control his pain by non-narcotic means.

I told Dr. L that, actually, I couldn't do very much about his pain because it was an organic pain, but that I would do all that I could possibly do; that I would do every bit that was humanly possible. So I first acknowledged that there was not very much that I could do—I'd better acknowledge my limitations. Dr. L knew he had organic pain; he knew he had cancer; he knew it was metastases; he knew he was dying. He knew that no man has power over death, and so I acknowledged my general helplessness. But I added that I would do everything I possibly could do—that I would extend every possible effort to help him.

I began by explaining time distortion to him. I explained how time can seem very long or very short. I pointed out that when he had an attack of stabbing pain it seemed to last for hours, while the brief moments of freedom from pain seemed all too short. Then I suggested that we'd better make the period of pain very, very short, and the period of freedom from pain very, very long—by using time distortion. Dr. L thought that was a good idea.

Next I pointed out that when you have anything wrong with you organically, you not only have (1) the organic pain itself, but you have (2) your psychological awareness of that pain, and you have (3) your own personality reaction to the pain. I reiterated: "So, actually, you have (1) organic pain; you have (2) your psychological reaction to that pain which intensifies and increases and enlarges the organic pain experience; and then you have (3) your personality reaction to your total situation, which makes you all the more sensitive to the organic pain and to your psychological reaction as well."

Now Dr. L could follow that reasoning, and so I suggested that he limit his pain just to the actual, organic pain. Just that and no more. You can take a needle and prick your finger intentionally in order to study the sensation of the needle prick, and you notice how easy it is to localize the needle prick. You feel the prick, but it is a very transient sensation. However, that needle prick would last for a long time if your big brother were pricking you with the needle to tease you.

Dr. L became interested in that idea as well, so I was able to cut down the organic pain to just that objective organic pain. But as soon as I started cutting down the organic pain just to the organic pain, I knew that you also can cut down organic pain by minimizing your response to it. You see, in organic pain situations you have neurosynapses that are transmitting the pain. Through hypnosis you can spread those synapses apart—like sparks jumping a gap—until you have your synapses spread so wide apart that you get a jumping of the thing. At that point a certain maximal pain stimulation is necessary in order for the person to sense the pain.

As soon as Dr. L's pain began to lessen through these measures, he became decidedly susceptible to hypnotic anesthesia. I had built up the entire situation with my acknowledgement of the organic, of the psychological reaction to the organic, and of the personality reaction to the organic. Then I started limiting the pain components to the organic and inducing a hypnotic anesthesia by bringing about those peculiar neuro-psycho-physiological responses that caused a separation of the neural synapses in the sensory nerves.

> Eds: Today we would recognize these "neuro-psycho-physiological responses that cause a separation of the neural synapses in the sensory nerves" as a metaphor for real

changes that are brought about in neurotransmitters and the neuroendocrinal system by suggestion.[6]

The result was that Dr. L tended to have little or no pain during the day. The pain he did have during the day tended to be rather brief, with long periods of time in which he was completely free from pain. I would go over in the evening around six o'clock; I would return about ten o'clock; and I would return again about eleven or half past eleven in order to ensure a peaceful night's sleep for him. This lasted until all his grandchildren and children arrived, at which point he had a long, delightful talk with each and every member of his family. His viewpoint was that he was going to die; he might as well visit with each family member and have a thoroughly good visit. It would exhaust him, he knew, but he might as well visit with everyone, even if it did exhaust him—even if it did cut short his life by an hour or a day.

After he had had a completely satisfactory visit with all his children and grandchildren, he rested up for one day and then the pain became unbearable; he lapsed into a coma and died. But he did have about two weeks of decidedly easy going before his death.

Pain Control in Cancer

Implication and a Behavioral Syllogism to "Prove" Hypnotic Pain Reduction: Dissociation in Somnambulistic Trance

I can think of another example of this problem of organic lesions. The patient had a carcinoma of the uterus with metastases all through her abdomen, her hipbone, and so on. Her surgeon had told her that she had about a month to live. The woman spent her days and nights sitting on the edge of her bed with extreme bladder urgency as a result of the metastases. She would start to doze off, and then immediately rouse up again.

She got her rest sitting on the edge of that bed, suffering from great pain, with just a wink of sleep now and then. She could never lay down for more than five minutes at a time.

Now this situation had been going on for two weeks, and her husband and two daughters were all exhausted from sitting there beside Mother to keep her from falling when she would doze off to sleep. The surgeon wanted to know if I would try hypnosis. In the same breath he said that it was useless to try, because morphine hadn't helped; Demerol hadn't helped; he didn't know if anything could help; therefore it would be useless to try hypnosis.

I went out to see the woman. She was at home, for she insisted on dying at home, and I raised with her the question of hypnosis. She said she didn't know whether or not she believed in hypnosis. I told her it was a perfectly good and sound tool. She had had a ninth-grade education; her husband had had a ninth-grade education; her 19-year-old daughter had graduated high school; and her 17-year-old daughter was completing high school. So I told her that if she didn't believe in hypnosis, perhaps the best way to find out if it were any good would be to have her daughters go to the library and look it up in the *Encyclopaedia Britannica*. I already had scanned the room and had spotted a different encyclopedia on the bookshelf, so I knew they respected encyclopedias; but their encyclopedia did not have an article on hypnosis. (Besides, I was a bit selfish about the *Britannica*—you'll see why in a few moments.)

The mother said she would think it over, and that she would send her daughters to the library to read the *Encyclopaedia Britannica's* article on hypnosis. Next, I told the daughter that I was the author of the hypnosis article (my motives are revealed), and she had better verify that. So I established my prestige with both the daughter and the mother—after all, a man who has written an article for an encyclopedia really ought to know his stuff.

I returned a week later and the mother said she was very glad her daughters had read that article, and that she would be willing to cooperate. But how could hypnosis really make her feel better? She didn't expect to live. She would just like one night's sleep—just one night of restful sleep before she died. I pointed out to her that I would have to do something that she might not understand, but that I could do it first with her daughters. I suggested that the 19-year-old daughter be a hypnotic subject for me. She agreed.

I began by suggesting that the daughter develop an intense pain in her knee, underneath her dress. A pain in her knee underneath her dress. Where was mother's cancer? Cancer of the uterus—underneath the dress. Daughter has a pain underneath the dress. The daughter actually hallucinated rather severe pain, and Mother didn't like that at all. Mother didn't understand. I told her that she wouldn't understand. I didn't want her to understand. I pointed out that even though that pain was in Daughter's knee, under Daughter's dress, that I could suggest that it slowly disappear and reappear in the other knee; and, of course, it did. The daughter was an excellent hypnotic subject. The transfer of pain from one knee to the other impressed Father who was observing, as well as Younger Daughter. It also thoroughly impressed Mother.

Next I asked the daughter to experience severe enough pain that she would want to cry, but that she would try to control her tears. And Daughter proceeded to hallucinate severe pain, and you could tell from her facial contortions that she was about to cry. She did shed a few tears. Mother didn't like that, but I told her Daughter would be glad to have that pain to teach Mother. So Mother let me go ahead, and I removed the pain, which showed Mother that I could start with her knees. Mother could also understand that I could start with her shoulders and her neck, and that I could bring about the convergence of increasing anesthesia, an increasing freedom from pain. She had seen her daughter literally shedding tears from pain. It was hallucinated pain, but Mother didn't understand that. All she knew was that the daughter she shortly was never to see again was having pain. It was very, very painful to Mother: seeing her daughter suffer pain was adding, psychologically, to her own pain. I relieved that pain by freeing the daughter of pain, and so Mother could recognize that she also could have freedom from pain.

You see, it is your willingness to recognize a total situation.

Never restrict your understanding just to a tooth, just to a cancerous spot, but direct your understanding to the total situation. To reiterate my line of reasoning: *Daughter suffering pain would be painful to Mother; I could relieve Daughter's pain; therefore I could relieve Mother's pain.* I could start with the knee. I had already done so with the daughter. Starting with the knee implied that I could just as well start with the shoulders, with the neck; and so I suggested the possibility of lying down on the bed and discovering all of the feelings of sleep that had been forgotten because of pain.

"Now what are the feelings of sleep? What are the feelings of your right hand as you lie flat on your back with your hand resting on the sheet? What are those feelings?" Mother began remembering and recalling those feelings. She wasn't thinking about the feeling of pain and distress in her bladder that gave her a sense of urinary urgency. "What is the feeling in the back of the left hand as you fall asleep?" I wanted to fixate her attention on the back of the hand; I wanted to focus her attention on the back of her right hand, the back of her left hand, the back of her heel, the back of her head, the back of her shoulders, the back of the calf of her leg. You can see how carefully I narrowed it down so that I could get a restful feeling in her buttocks, a restful feeling in the small of her back, a restful feeling in her knees, and that sense of sleepiness.

After reviving and recalling all the memories of restful sleep, I taught the mother how to walk into the bathroom. I stressed that she must remember how to walk to the bathroom at least every three hours—possibly every two-and-a-half hours, but really, honestly, I thought every three hours would be often enough. What Mother didn't realize, what the daughters didn't realize, what the father didn't realize, was that I was giving her a urinary frequency of every three hours—not every five minutes—but a definite three-hour frequency. I'd better go along with that cancer. Cancer had given her an almost continuous need to go to the bathroom. I'd better accept that bladder urgency, but I'd also better control it and make it a three-hour one.

Next I taught the mother how to go into a somnambulistic

trance, how to talk to her daughters while in this somnambulistic trance, and how to walk from one room to another. Why did I want the mother to walk? It was an utterly useless activity for her. She did not need the exercise. The walking was a useless expenditure of energy except for the walk to the bathroom. But, you know, if you can walk—that implies you can sit down; if you can sit down—that implies you can lie down; and so I had her walk to imply that if I could tell her to walk, I could tell her to lie down and go to sleep. (I knew she wouldn't recognize consciously the psychological implications of the walking.)

The mother developed a nice anesthesia. She would have her three-hour urgency and she was always glad to go to the bathroom. She took her fruit juices along to make it a worthwhile trip, and she had her pain every time she went to the bathroom, because I knew she had better have some pain that she recognized. So she had pain during urination—she was convinced that, as a cancer patient, you always have pain with it, and I went along with that idea. That was her understanding and I'd better accept it; I'd better abide by it. And so she had pain every time she went to the bathroom. She emptied her bladder, she had pain, she left the bathroom. She could go back to bed or she could go back to that reclining chair; *she could go into a somnambulistic trance and talk to her daughters; she could come out of the somnambulistic trance but leave one part of her body in a trance state by the matter of dissociation.* In short, she could do a lot of things.

Any organic problem can be approached effectively. I cited Robert with his split lip. I have cited the two cancer cases as extreme examples of pathology. I could cite another cancer case in which I taught the patient a somnambulistic dissociated state. For a month the patient had a completely delightful time visiting with all the family, and then suddenly, in the middle of a visit, she lapsed into a coma and died. But she had enjoyed that month or five weeks of living.

The same approach applies to any organic problem: you accept it; you recognize all of its implications; you never fight against it; and you use it in a way that is to the patient's advantage. You never try to deny it or dispute it or contradict it.

The Use of Language in Hypnosis

The Importance of Understanding the Meanings and Associations of Words Used to Influence Psychological and Organic Life

During the intermission a question was put to me: "Are you aware of the way in which you use your words?" I certainly am, and I want to emphasize the importance of that awareness to all of you.

In hypnosis you are going to use words to influence the psychological life of your patient today; you are going to use words to influence his organic life today; you are going to also influence his psychological and organic life twenty years from now. So you had better know what you are saying. You had better be willing to reflect upon the words you use, to wonder what their meanings are, and to seek out and understand their many associations.

I can recall one of my most embarrassing experiences as a medical student. I had been reading about fingernails—about how one can look at fingernails and recognize that the length of growth in them can tell one something about illness. I had read about how a ridge can develop across all the fingernails when a person has a severe illness.

Well, we had one female medical student in the class, and I happened to look at her fingernails, and every one of them showed a ridge across it. I said promptly, "When were you sick last?" At this point I learned to understand thoroughly the meaning of words, because she looked at me in such a horrified fashion—she really was ready to swing at me. I managed to recover, and said, "Was it pneumonia, because I see those fingernail ridges?" She looked down at her fingernails and realized that I was just a simple country kid who didn't know any better than to talk that way.*

---

*Editors' Note: In those days being "sick" was a euphemism for having a menstrual period.

Since that experience I have been trying to watch my words—to understand their meanings. When you see a woman dying of cancer of the uterus you ought to know that it is pain that is underneath the dress; and if you want to teach her something about that pain you had better start in some simple way with the pain under the dress. And if you are using the dying woman's daughter as a subject, you had better use the daughter's knee for a gradual approach, because the daughter's knee is a rather sacred area, and yet it is a safe teaching area, too. It is your willingness to examine and recognize your words.

Hypnotic Anesthesia and Analgesia

Indirect Apposition of Opposites to Effect Dental Anesthesia: Shifting Hyperasthesia from Mouth to Hand

Next I have been requested to discuss the technique of hypnotic anesthesia and analgesia. No matter what you are suggesting to a patient—whether it is an anesthesia or analgesia, a relaxation, an attitude toward one's mother-in-law, or whatever—it is your task to present an idea so that the person listens to you; so that the person understands you; so that the person knows that you are talking about a particular subject, and so that the person is willing to listen and understand. You need to recognize that you approach different subjects in different ways, and that the technique you choose must be based upon your awareness of the totality of the problem.

I'll give you an example. A patient went in to visit a dental friend of mine and said; "I need a lot of dental work done on my mouth. I am a good hypnotic subject, and I want hypnosis used. In college I always volunteered, but I have never had any dentistry done under hypnosis. I need a lot done now, so I decided to have dental anesthesia."

The dentist was delighted, and set about producing a hand anesthesia with transfer from the hand to the mandible. The patient developed a perfectly beautiful anesthesia of the hand, but he couldn't transfer it to his mandible. So the dentist tried the other hand, and presto, a beautiful anesthesia there—but he couldn't transfer it. Next he suggested that the anesthesia radiate from the right hand to the left hand to the mandible. No good. The patient could develop anesthesia of the foot, of the leg, of the belly, of the shoulder blades, of the hands—but no anesthesia of his mouth or face. He just couldn't.

Another dentist tried and failed, and so the question arose as to what could be done. The patient was brought to the Hypnotic Study Club and I was asked how I would approach such a problem. The patient had an extremely sensitive mouth, there was no doubt about that. He was ready to jump out of his chair if you just touched his lip. He emphatically could not develop an anesthesia of the mouth. I explained that I would use the same approach to this patient's hypersensitivity that I had employed many years ago when I was a kid at home on the farm.

One blizzardy day in mid-winter, my father tried to pull a calf into the barn. The calf braced itself staunchly against my father's effort; neither one was making any progress, and I stood there and laughed at both of them. My father said, "If you are so smart, you pull the calf in yourself, or at least help me to do it!" I said, "I'll pull the calf in alone," whereupon I took hold of the calf, grabbed it by the tail, and tried to pull it *out* of the barn. That calf showed me: *it* dragged *me* into the barn, exactly where we wanted it! So that was the basic technique I suggested.

> Eds: In another version of this same story which Erickson told later in life, his father was still trying to pull the calf into the barn while Milton pulled on its tail. The calf in this version trampled over Dad as it pulled Milton into the barn. In this version the situation presents a double bind to the calf, who chooses the lesser of two evils (it would rather move into the barn than have its tail pulled on), which, of course, was what Erickson wanted.

More specifically, I told the two dentists to practice the following on two volunteer patients who were present: "Go into the other room and produce hyperasthesia of their hands, and really produce a hyperasthesia, and work out a good technique on them." And so they took two volunteer patients into another room and worked out a good hyperasthesia technique. Next I told them, "Take your patient who cannot develop an anesthesia of the mouth and develop a thorough-going hyperasthesia of his left hand. Really build it up until you can tell him, 'Just to breathe on it will make you wince with pain.' Really build it up."

Well, the patient was rather astonished to discover that he developed a hyperasthesia of his hand, and in the process, drained all of the hyperasthesia from his mouth into that hand. You see, the patient's thinking was essentially this: "I've got a very sensitive mouth; I've got hyperasthesia. I'm going to keep that hyperasthesia, and there is nothing you can do about it." All I did was move the hyperasthesia down here to the hand where the dentist would have no cause to touch upon it, and so the patient had his anesthesia and his hyperasthesia as well. [He got his cake and ate it, too!]

Habit Problems

Utilizing Confrontation to Evoke Agressiveness in the Control of Organic Spasms: "Sit on It!"

Let's consider next those unnecessary habits that people develop—that winking of one eye or that pulling on one ear or that twisting of one finger every time you talk to them—until you could say, "Have the darned thing amputated!" There are all kinds of annoying little things that people get into the habit of doing, and they do them so automatically. They are unaware of those habits.

I can think of a rather extreme example. A patient came to me who had had an encephalitis with a resulting spastic paralysis. Her left arm waved in all directions whenever she sat down and talked to you; and her left leg kept her left hand in erratic company waving around all the time she talked to you; and it was so disagreeable to try to talk to her. She asked me if I could use hypnosis on her to improve matters.

I pointed out that there was an organic basis for the waving of her left leg, and that there was an organic basis for the spasmodic movements of her left hand. I looked the girl over very, very carefully, and then I questioned her thoroughly. The girl was a decidedly aggressive person, a rather antagonistic person, and she was rather hostile in giving her history. She told me that I really should get to work on cutting down her erratic movements instead of taking so much history. All I needed to know was that she had had the encephalitis, and why take the additional history since my neurological and psychological training was sufficient to allow me to figure the rest out for myself. She saw no need for me to go into too many details.

My feeling was that any college girl who was majoring in psychology and who was able to express her hostility so freely—she could really dish it out—could probably take it as well. So, I said: "You are rather hostile and aggressive. Can you take it as well as dish it out?" And she said: "Why, certainly I can. Don't you think I have learned to do that?"

With that clear reply I proceeded: "Well, I see no excuse for you waving your foot and no excuse for you waving your hand, because you can take your right leg and drape it over your left leg, and the weight of your right leg will hold that left leg down; and then your fanny is big enough so that you can sit on your left hand and hold it down; and then we can talk about how you might correct the habit."

This woman now has her doctorate in psychology. About a year ago we went out to dine in a restaurant. We walked in together, and my limp was obvious. The waiter noticed it, and he took my cane very nicely; in fact, he helped me take off my overcoat as well. But he left my companion to take off her own coat. Then he brought my coat and cane to me, and I asked him, "Didn't you notice that the lady limps also, and didn't you notice that she needed a little help with her coat, too?" He looked at me in a puzzled way and said that he hadn't noticed it, but he had noticed mine.

She still waves her arm a little bit, but you seldom notice it. Now what had I done? I had simply directed her attention to the fact that she could do something abut her hand waving by parking her fanny on it. It wasn't a polite, a thoughtful, a courteous way to phrase the matter, but yet, with her, it was.

Treating Tics via Reframing

Questions to Fixate Attention, Heighten Consciousness, and Provoke Discovery

What do you do with patients who twist your ear off? You need to get their attention, and, above all, you need to get them to recognize that they do carry out those habitual acts. You need to get that patient with the winking right eye to discover that he does wink that right eye of his too many times in the course of an hour; and you need to raise the question of tics with him. You do not raise the question of *does* he wink his eye, but you raise the question of *what muscles is he employing* in the winking of his eye: is it the masseter muscle, or is it the tubular vandibular muscle, or possibly the orbicularis ocularis muscle, or is it the risus sardonicus muscle?

What are you doing? You are asking him questions in medical terminology, and he knows darned well that he doesn't understand which muscles you are talking about, but he does wish that you would speak ordinary language. And in that wishing he is really asking you to identify the muscle that closes the eye—or is it the muscle that works on the upper part of the jawbone, or the muscle that does the chewing, or possibly the muscle that lifts the corner of the mouth into a sneer when you really don't like somebody's hat? The patient is inviting you to drop that medical terminology, and, of course, you also want to drop it, but when he invites you to drop it, he is also inviting you to discuss that functional tic. *He is wide open to a discovery.* Does he blink his eye once a minute, twice a minute? How aware is he of the movement? Whereabouts does he first get the feeling—is it in front of the ear, or is it right at the edge of his nose, or underneath the eyebrow, or in the upper lid? In other words, you are asking the patient with a tic to thoroughly discuss his tic, and you are also asking him to fragment that tic.

You would approach patients with functional tics of a dental origin in the same way: you get their attention, and you get them wishing that you'd talk to them in a language that they can understand. The very simplicity of your attitude is the key.

> Eds: In this process of asking questions and getting the patient to wish the therapist would use ordinary language, we can again divine the origins of Erickson's beginning use of "shifting frames of reference," or *reframing*. When the patient is not conscious of the eye winking, it may become an autonomous, unconscious habit. The questions about which muscles are used raises the patient's consciousness and introduces new experiential variables into the habit situation which the patient can then learn how to control. This introduction of new, controllable experiential variables makes this reframing vastly more effective in habit problems than the reframing described earlier in which pain was simply "nullified, contradicted, or otherwise shifted out of the focus of attention." It thus becomes apparent that *different types of psychological problems will require different forms of reframing*. This is indeed a new therapeutic approach that requires a great deal of research in both laboratory and clinical settings.

Indirect Hypnotic Induction Techniques

Fixation of Attention via Eye Contact and Vocal Tone Versus Formal Techniques: Trance Without Awareness of It

The question I have failed to discuss so far is when do I induce a trance and what technique do I use in inducing it? How many people in the audience are in a trance from listening to me at the present time? I can see that there are a number of you in deep trances.

You see, when I talk to a patient in my office I fixate his gaze on me, and I talk to him in such a fashion that he knows I am talking to him, he knows that I want him to listen, that I want him to hear me, and that I am not the least bit interested in the noise outside of my office—in the airplane overhead, in the cars driving down the street, in the bird in the backyard that's singing. *I am talking just to him, and I am holding his attention. He feels fixated and he feels rigid, but the softness of my voice and the directness of my gaze compel all of his attention to me, and so he is in a trance state. That is the technique I usually employ, because I don't like to waste time in a formal technique of suggesting,* "Now you uncross your legs and you put your feet flat on the floor. Now you lean back and you fixate your gaze." It takes too much time, and I have a lot of work to do with that patient, so I simply talk. I don't know how rapidly the patient can learn, how readily he can understand, or how much value the hypnosis is going to have for him. With some patients it is effective very rapidly, with others it works more slowly. Patients need to take their time, and it isn't important that they realize that they have been in a trance—their unconscious will know it.

Habit Problems

Treating Bruxism via Conditioned Substitution: "A Habit You Give Up in a Hurry"

In addition to the functional tic I have discussed, there is this matter of bruxism which gives you the opportunity of using a different kind of technique. The adult or the child comes to you with bruxism—grinding of the teeth. One technique I have used with adults is a rather simple technique. All adults can take pride in this matter of falling asleep the minute their heads hit the pillow. Or they can take pride in falling asleep without a pillow the minute they put their heads down. That is the safer way, because so many people don't put their heads on pillows. So you don't give a posthypnotic suggestion to fall asleep "when your head hits the pillow" but "when you put your head down." And so you talk to your adult bruxism patient about "how nice it is to fall asleep instantly when you put your head down—the instant you are ready to go to sleep it is so delightful to go sound asleep into a deep physiological sleep." Having built up the patient's legitimate narcissistic pride in going into a sound physiological sleep, you can then point out to him: "And whenever you go into sound physiological sleep, there is the possibility that this night or the next night, that this week or the next week, you will grind your teeth. But from now on, whenever that does occur... [material lost in recording]. As soon as you have made that bruxism unpleasant and inconvenient the person will quit doing it, and that is what you want.

You can also use the technique of conditioning the bruxism patient to awaken whenever teeth grinding occurs. You point out that it is a very nice thing to have a good grip of the hand, and people are so lazy about exercising—they always skip their calisthenics: "Every time you grind your teeth, you exercise your grip until you get a really good grip." This is especially effective with little children. You really let them take pride in their exercise, pride in the strength of their grip.

What are you doing? You are conditioning the bruxism to exercise, and you are giving the patient a favorable attitude toward the bruxism; but at the same time you are making the habit inconvenient, because who wants to wake up in the middle of the night and get a perfectly good grip? The patient may postpone the gripping exercise until the morning, after he has had a night's sleep, but you are still conditioning him to awaken.

With a small child you can reinforce these suggestions by tying sponge rubber in the hand and endowing that sponge rubber with nice properties: "It will help your fingers to open and enable you to get a very strong arm." And I can brag about my own grip, and I can show the child the play of my muscles under the skin, and I can point out that I grip my cane a great deal: "I have a wonderful grip in my left hand," and the child can listen and know that I am talking sincerely and honestly. He can be glad that he can exercise his hand and not have to carry a cane to get that good grip. He is agreeing that one shouldn't have to have bad habits such as bruxism or limping to get a good grip. So you are generalizing the total understandings of the child or the adult.

Another approach is to condition the person to the idea that every time he grinds his teeth he will awaken, and that he can go to sleep with gum tucked in between his cheek and his teeth. You explain that he must learn to sleep that way so that every time he grinds his teeth he will slip that gum in between his teeth, chew it for a while, then carefully tuck it back against his cheek and go back to sleep. And so he chews the gum, and you have transformed the bruxism into a gum-chewing habit. Who wants a gum-chewing habit in the middle of the night? That is a habit you give up in a hurry, and again it is making the bruxism habit a most inconvenient activity.

The same approach is effective for fingernail biting or thumb sucking: *You transform bad habits in character [by altering their behavioral value or function], or you transform them in the patient's subjective experience by making them unpleasant, inconvenient, or faulty.*

Group Hypnotherapy

Special Personality and Therapeutic Considerations

Group therapy is the next issue I want to discuss. In working with groups you ought to bear in mind, first and foremost, the matter of whether or not your own personality is suited for dealing with a group. Too many professionals attempt to conduct group therapy and then discover that it just doesn't work. [They're not sure why, and in evaluating what went wrong] they often overlook the important question: Is their own personality such that they can work with a group?

As a therapist I personally don't know how to work with a group. I can recognize that Dr. A can work beautifully with groups; he's got that kind of a personality. I don't know how to describe that kind of a personality in exact terms, but the professional who is considering group work should raise the question first of all: "Am I the kind of a person who can do therapy with a group?" I know, for example, that I can teach in a group situation: I can teach with a large group; I can teach with a small group; I can teach with one person. But I don't seem to be able to do group therapy.

In addition to having the right kind of personality for group work, realize also that it is your job to provide an orientation for the group. Sometimes the orientation for the group is yourself; sometimes the orientation is someone else. For example, in hypnotic group work for pregnant women, your first step is to demonstrate hypnosis by using one of the women as a subject. How do you choose which woman? My thinking would be: I would like to use a simple, straightforward, unaffected, utterly delightful primipara*—a woman who is responsive to hypnosis, who is so unaffected, so sweet, and so simple. I don't mean unintelligent. I just mean unaffected, simple, and direct. She is the type to have as the center of the group. Why? Because you know every multipara in that group is going to like that girl. They aren't going to be jealous of her; they aren't going to feel catty toward her; and so you have a nice, central orientation, and all the other women in the group can look at her and not be jealous of her and not feel in competition with her. She is a primipara, and they are all second or multiparas; and they certainly are going to be willing to learn everything that she knows, because they know a lot more than she does. She is a primipara, and even if she does know more about hypnosis than they do, it is they who know about the really vital issue—that of childbirth. So, you create a situation that is entirely acceptable to all the group members, and with that safe young mother, you can set the example of this learning and that learning.

Another important point to keep in mind is the following: Always in group therapy you stress the separateness of learning for each patient. One patient shows good hand levitation with the right hand, but someone else shows good levitation with the left hand; some show an early closing of the eyelids; and others show an early loss of the swallowing reflex. So in your group

---

Editors' Note: Primipara is an obstetrical term for a woman who is giving birth for the first time; *multipara* refers to a woman who has given birth to more than two children.

situation you always define the individual as an individual, but against the background of the total group: "You are the one with the early loss of the swallowing reflex, while he is the one with the early right hand levitation." I am just using very recognizable examples. Naturally, you have to utilize whatever behaviors are being dealt with in your particular group situation. If you are doing group psychotherapy it will be one matter. If you are using a group situation to condition a number of dental patients on how to wear their dentures without gagging, that is another matter. But the point is that *you always define the individual as an individual, and you always define him as a member of the group.*

DEMONSTRATION:

Evoking and Utilizing Ideomotor Head Movements for Subject Selection in Audiences

E: Will the person who feels awfully cold please stand up? There is one of you there in the draft. Will you please stand up? Please stand up.

It's all in knowing where the draft is. I singled that out because it would leave time for thinking and feeling. Now, I am going to put my next question to the subject.

A Double-Bind Question to Ratify Trance

E: If you know that you are in a trance, nod your head this way. If you don't know it, shake your head this way.

> Eds: Here Erickson demonstrates a very slow, slight head nodding for yes and head shaking for no. If the audience member responds with a spontaneous nodding or shaking, it is a ratification of the existence of trance because that type of spontaneous slow movement is itself a characteris-

tic of trance. If the subject shakes the head no, it simply means she is in trance without awareness of it.

She is in pretty good trance. It is eleven o'clock, on the nose. Notice the tremendous interest of the group in just what I am trying to do. The question is, how about a quick test, now, for those in a trance—right now, in the audience? Dr. Brody, will you tell the audience what you said to me?

Dr. Brody: Previous to the 10:30 session, Dr. Erickson asked me if I had noticed how many audience members were in a trance. I knew some were, but I did not know the exact number. So at eleven o'clock I looked the audience over for my own recognition. I thought there were sixteen to seventeen people here in a moderate to deep trance at eleven o'clock.

E: Right now there is one person still in a very, very deep trance, but of course that person really doesn't know that the self can go into a deep trance and listen to a lecture. But that person is still maintaining that trance and will keep on maintaining that trance.

Dr. Brody: I might say there is one doctor here in a nice trance, and he says he can *never* go into a trance. Harold, I am talking about you. Nobody could ever hypnotize him. Put your hand up, Harold.

Facilitating Learning and Recall

Utilizing Audience Hypnosis in the Retention and Comprehension of Lecture Material

E: [Talking to Margie, the woman in the draft] Do you mind being in a trance? You can listen to me all day in a trance. Did you know that?

Margie (M): No.

E: You didn't know it. That is right, Margie. You have been in a trance throughout my entire lecture, and I am awfully glad you were, because Dr. Brody has asked me a question. It is a question I have encountered many, many times. If you want to, Margie, I would like to have you sit down with a tape recorder sometime in the future and, just for the fun of it, recall my lecture. Go into a trance state, recall my lecture, and dictate it into a tape recorder. Dictate, let us say, what I said the first part of the morning, what I said the latter part of the morning. Now I know you do not have the professional training to cover all the material, but I do know that next week you can dictate into a tape recorder your recollection of your understandings of the things I have said, and you can do it very, very beautifully, and very adequately. And you can do it in accord with your own understanding.

In exactly the same way, every one of you professionals in the audience could sit down next week or next month to a tape recorder and dictate your recollections to a surprising extent. Another thing you might discover is that you could play back your dictated recording a month later and, without going into a trance, recall what is going to be said next; and you could sit there listening but knowing just what the next sentence will be, verbatim.

Characteristics of Spontaneous Audience Trance

Now, I have been talking to the audience while Margie has been standing here in a trance. Do you see how utterly rigid she is, how her eyes do not blink, how her hands remain that way, how there is an absence of the swallowing reflex? She is just as immobile as can be. And there are quite a number of you that I notice are in the same state—sixteen of you, I think, is a good count. And there are others in the audience who now and then went into a trance, and then came out of it. Why? Because there is that willingness to listen and to go into a trance.

Trance and Learning Without Awareness

Structuring Unexpected Trance Situations to Facilitate Unconscious Learning

Margie expected me to put her into a trance later today. She didn't expect to go into a trance so early this morning. I knew that she was likely not to have that expectation. *That is why I often induce trances in my office by just talking to patients about the things they are interested in, and without telling them that they are in a trance.* They might expect me to waste a good fifteen minutes on a hand levitation technique, whereas this way they can listen, they can learn, and they can understand.

One can also make use of the type of situation Margie has just demonstrated so beautifully in experimental situations. When I was teaching at Wayne University College of Medicine and at Wayne County General Hospital, I would teach my residents in psychiatry how to go into a trance. Then I would take up a case history and discuss it at very great length—with some of the residents in a trance and some of the residents not in a trance. A month later I would institute an examination in my usual, unpredictable, inexcusable fashion. I would simply say, "I have decided to give you a test today. I would like to have you summarize your understandings of Cases X, Y, Z." The residents who had been awake during my experimental lecture a month ago would say, "Well, okay, but we haven't reviewed it recently"; and the residents who had been in a trance during my lecture would say, "But we have never had that case—you never discussed it with us—we don't know a thing about it!" And I would say: "Well, some of you know about it. You are all equally responsible for understanding the material, and if some of you do know it, it must be because I assigned it to you in the past; and if some of you failed to get your assignment, that is just your tough luck. There is the paper, there is the chair, and there is the desk. Sit down and start working."

Those who had been in a trance would sit down, and after a few minutes' time a thought would come into their mind, and then another thought, and another—and soon they would be writing away. After I had pulled this trick on them a couple of times they did not fret about the exam. They knew their unconscious would recognize the material: "This is the time for me to put up and make available to my conscious mind the knowledge that I have acquired unconsciously."

So I could only pull that startling, shocking experience on students about twice. Thereafter they knew that their unconscious would measure up. And that is something all of you need to know: *your unconscious can learn without letting you know it is learning; but at the right time and in the right situation it will shove up into the conscious mind the essential knowledge.*

Posthypnotic Suggestion for Appetite Control

E: Now, Margie, I am going to offer you a suggestion, and it is going to be a posthypnotic suggestion for the entire group. We are going to lunch. I want you to enjoy your meal fully and completely, and to really enjoy it. And for those in the audience who need to eat a small portion, I want them to enjoy that small portion so completely that it satisfies their appetite as if it were ten times that size. In other words, I want those who need to watch their diets to enjoy their food very completely—just a small portion.

All right, Margie, sit down and wake yourself, wide awake—wide awake. Hi, Margie! It is time for a break.

Autohypnosis in Everyday Life

Following Circuitous Associations Straight to the Goal: Mrs. Erickson's Forgotten Task

I want to cite an example from personal experience on this matter of unconscious learning and unconscious memory. I use autohypnosis; Mrs. Erickson uses autohypnosis. I will cite one of Mrs. Erickson's experiences.

One Sunday afternoon Mrs. Erickson was reading the Sunday

paper. The family was scattered around the house, and all of a sudden Mrs. Erickson got up and said, "There is something I ought to do this afternoon." I said, "Well, what is it?" and she answered, "I don't know, but I've got to do it this afternoon." I said, "You'll waste a lot of time if you want to try to figure it out." She said, "I wasn't going to waste any time. I am going to let my unconscious do it for me." Then she smiled and added, "You know, I washed yesterday. I think I'll go out to the garage and see if the washing machine is still there."

Now really, who would steal a washing machine? That was a completely ridiculous, silly, purposeless statement. But she went on out to the garage and looked and the washing machine was still there. She looked at it, and then she happened to notice that the work bench at the end of the garage was all messed up. Allan had been working there, and he never hangs up a single tool; and she made a mental note that Allan ought to straighten up the work bench.

Having done those monumental tasks—finding out that the washing machine was still there, and noting, incidentally, that the work bench was messy—she went over to the other side of the backyard and looked to see if the fish pond were still there. It was. Nobody had stolen the fish pond, and so she wandered back into the house. Now easily, casually, indifferently, she came in through the back door. As she came through the back door she happened to get a full view of a certain bookcase; and naturally the books were out of line, so she wandered over and straightened up the books, accidentally dropping one on the floor. She picked it up, read the title, smiled to herself, walked into the other room, and said: "Allan, here is a book for you to read. Your father and I decided several years ago that when you got far enough along in high school you would understand things well enough to be able to read this book. Here it is. You will enjoy reading it." And she handed him the book. Now there was Mrs. Erickson doing the task she had set out to do but couldn't quite remember.

What is the background of her recollection? On Friday afternoon Allan had come home from school bringing his grades. We had looked at them casually. They were reasonably good, and that is all we did about his grades. They were reasonably good.

Then Friday evening passed, Saturday passed, Saturday evening, Sunday morning, Sunday afternoon. Mrs. Erickson had something to do. What was it? So she got up to see if the washing machine was still there. The washing machine uses water. It very definitely uses water. The work bench. Allan's work bench was messed up. Something undone by Allan—something that needed to be done. Over to the fish pond... that is a body of water. It is still there, there were fish in it, and she looked down in the water. A body of water with small bodies in it. Next, she came into the house, happened to spot a particular bookcase with the books out of order, and went over to straighten things out. Accidentally or unconsciously she knocked a certain book down. The title of the book was, *The Man Who Never Was.* It was a book about that spy story of World War II where a man's dead body was dropped into the Atlantic Ocean, washed ashore in Spain, found, and turned over to the Germans. The Germans searched the body, found complete plans for the invasion of Italy, and modified their campaign. That was how the allies caught the Germans off guard. A tremendously important thing. The body that fell into a body of water.

Now Mrs. Erickson and I had both read that book several years before and had decided that Allan should read it when he was old enough to understand it. His marks from high school on Friday afternoon had indicated that he was old enough and far enough through high school to understand the book. [But the memory of that decision to give Allan the book at the right time was still in Mrs. Erickson's unconscious.] So she went about recovering it in a purely unconscious way, by building up associations—the washing machine with water, the work bench, Allan, Something undone, the body of water (the fish pond) with bodies in it (fish), the bookcase and the book—and that was it! Mrs. Erickson walked into the room and handed the book to Allan.

She was using her unconscious; she was just following whatever associations came into her mind. Too many people try to use their unconscious in too direct a way by forcing themselves to adhere to the belief that they must proceed directly to the goal. I wonder how much time Mrs. Erickson would have spent had she sat there and consciously pondered, "Now what was it;

what did I need to do; what should I do? There's got to be something. I know there is something." Where would she have gotten? She gave herself the freedom to follow her unconscious. You always need to respect your unconscious.

Erickson's Unfinished Manuscript

The Provisional Role of the Conscious Mind in Relation to the Unconscious

I had a couple of hours to spend one day, and Mrs. Erickson said to me: "The publisher is yammering his head off about that manuscript. Why don't you finish it?" I said: "Well, I've got two hours. I might as well." So I closed my office door and decided to go into a trance. I knew very well that if I went into a trance I might write the manuscript, and I certainly could afford to use my unconscious in the writing of it. At the end of two hours I awakened. The patient who was scheduled for that time arrived, and I completed my day's work with never a thought about what had happened during those two hours.

The next week Mrs. Erickson said, "Did you finish that manuscript last week?" I answered, "That's right, I forgot about it completely." She said, "Did you work on it?" I said, "I don't know. Let's find it." I keep manuscripts in one of four places. I looked in all four places. No manuscript. Mrs. Erickson looked in all four places. No manuscript. She said, "I didn't misplace it." I said, "I probably did, let's forget about it. Let the publisher keep on suffering."

About a month later the patient came back for a check-up. As he entered the office I hauled out his case record—there was the lost manuscript. I looked at the manuscript, I looked at the patient. I realized that I could get another case history to add to that manuscript through this patient. My unconscious knew a month ago that I shouldn't write up that report for the publisher; it knew that I should wait until that patient came in who was due back in one month's time. So my unconscious hid the manuscript. I don't know what else I could have done with the two hours of time. Maybe I went into a physiological sleep. Maybe the trance allowed me to sit and analyze some of my case records, because I do a lot of my case record analysis in a trance. I think faster and more clearly in a trance than I do in the ordinary waking state.

You see, you make use of your unconscious. You need provide it only the time, place, and situation; and you bear in mind that your unconscious is just as bright as you are. In fact, it is a bit brighter than you are, because you are always handicapping yourself by your relationship to external reality. Your unconscious is much more concerned abut essential values. You get in trouble when you consciously try to interfere with your unconscious, and then your unconscious punishes you for interfering with the goodness of its work. *You provide the time, place, and situation, and then you let your unconscious select out of the 10,000 things you ought to do the thing that it considers most important for you to do.*

Problem-Solving Capacities of the Unconscious

Erickson's Clear, Creative Comics: Huey, Dewey, and Louie

There was a chapter that I just couldn't write for a certain paper. I couldn't figure out how to portray the illogic of one of my patients. I went into a trance wondering if I'd work on that case or another case, and I found out later that I had spent the time reading a whole bunch of comic books. I had used up the entire time reading a bunch of comic books.

The next opportunity I got to work on the paper I was perfectly content to do it in a waking state. I came to the difficult section I hadn't been able to portray, and, that's right, Huey, Dewey, Louie, and Donald Duck had paraphrased that very situation, that particular type of logic! My unconscious mind had sent me to the box of comic books and had me search through them until I had found the exact paraphrasing that I had wanted to use. In comic books, you have to make behaviors awfully, awfully clear, and sometimes the behaviors that are made clear are really extremely complex. And so I hadn't wasted my time reading those comic books.

The Case of the Blocked Artist

Utilizing the Unconscious Through Autohypnosis in Creative Work: Autonomous Ideomotor Movements in Trance

A friend of mind came to me and said, "For three years now I haven't had an artistic idea of any kind. I work eight hours a day and I haven't created a single piece of art. I blank out every time I start to think about artistic creation. I want to learn autohypnosis. I don't want anybody to hypnotize me. I want to learn autohypnosis." He flatly refused to be hypnotized, so the technique I gave him was to sit down for twenty minutes or so in his chair after his day's work and relax; just slump in the chair with his head down and enjoy the relaxation, and let his unconscious do as it pleased.

> Eds: This seems to be an example of how Erickson utilized the ultradian rhythm to facilitate autohypnosis even before its psychophysiological correlates were established in the laboratory.[7]

That visit took place in the last part of November. In January the man came to see me and said: "You know, I have been doing what you instructed me to do very regularly. I haven't missed a night. I get twenty minutes of relaxation, and sometimes even a half hour or an hour. I often wonder if I go into physiological sleep during that time, so I thought I'd come over and let you see how I relax." "What about your art?" I asked. "Well," he said, "I figured out a few things consciously. I've got a new piece of sculpturing that I am doing, but I'll talk to you about that later—but nothing has come out of my unconscious."

And he slumped down in his chair, and I watched his thumb which began doing something rather odd and peculiar, and I took pencil and paper and I graphed what his thumb was doing.

After about twenty minutes he roused up and said, "You see, I just relax. I keep my head down and I don't move. I just let my mind go blank, and I don't think I have learned anything about autohypnosis." And then he continued: "Now, concerning that

ERICKSON (VOL.2): LIFE REFRAMING IN HYPNOSIS

2:5 - 3:1 EMPHASISING PLEASURE
7:2 - 10:2 + 3 - 14:1
31:4

> DON'T LABOUR THE POINT YOU WANT TO MAKE. JUST MENTION IT ONCE IN PASSING.

JOHANN MICHAEL HAYDN.   Austria.   1737 – 1806.

Polonaise in C major.
Jorg Baumann – Cello.   Klaus Stoll – Double Bass.

piece of sculpture that I am working on: I have developed a new rhythm pattern that I am employing. I worked it out consciously. My unconscious had nothing to do with it. Let me have some paper and pencil and I will draw you a picture of the rhythm." And I said, "Will this picture of the rhythm be all right?", and I handed him my own drawing. He looked at it and said, "That is correct, but where did you get it?" I said, "It just came to me." He studied it and said, "That is exactly the rhythm that I worked out. It is a very unique pattern, but I wonder how you worked out a similar, unique pattern!" I sidestepped the question, and we talked on other subjects.

When he got home he finished up that particular piece of sculpture he had fully formed, like Minerva's spring, in his unconscious mind. Now it seemed that he had just one tremendous space of ideas coming up in the matter of painting and sculpturing. He has developed several new techniques, and he has every artistic idea. And his final statement to me was, "I guess I must have gone into an autohypnotic trance." That's right, he did. I watched him demonstrate that rhythm with his thumb, but everything else about him—the loss of reflexes, the immobility of his face, his unresponsiveness to the fact that I could rattle things on the desk, I could get up and cross the room, I could do anything and he remained oblivious to it—indicated that he was in a trance. In autohypnosis, you merely give yourself the opportunity of doing things with your unconscious.

Autohypnotic Techniques

Induction via a Hallucinated "Joe"; Trusting the Unconscious; Accepting Different Speeds and Styles of Learning in Autohypnosis

Any of you who want to use autohypnosis ought to sit down quietly and give yourself a chance. What kind of a technique can you use? One of the techniques that I have taught quite a number of college students interested in psychology is this: I have them sit down and look at my friend Joe sitting in that chair—the little man who isn't there—and I tell them to produce in Joe this hand levitation. I tell them to levitate Joe's hand until it touches his face, and to watch Joe close his eyes, take a deep breath, and go deep asleep. And so they use that technique in the privacy of their own homes. They sit down and imagine there is a chair over there with an imaginary man named Joe sitting in it, and they very carefully show Joe how to sit with his hands on his lap. And then they start suggesting hand levitation, eyelid closure, a deeper and deeper trance, and they go into their own trances. I usually have them try it once in my office to be sure they understand.

Now, there are psychology students who are tremendously interested in this approach. They haven't got any money for psychiatrists' fees, and why should I spend a lot of time teaching them something that they can learn very, very quickly? And so they sit there, and usually one experience is all that is necessary for them to go into a very satisfactory trance. Then the next thing to teach them after they are in a trance is to respect their own unconscious. And they've all found out that if they go into an autohypnotic trance, let us say, for the preordained purpose of studying geometry, they will wind up studying ancient history, or some other subject, because their unconscious minds will not take that kind of dictation. And so, one by one, they reach the understanding that when they go into a trance, they also must trust their own unconscious to pick the right things for them to do.

The last issue in this matter of autohypnosis is the willingness of the person to learn at his own speed. Why should Joe decide that he should learn at Anne's speed? In the first place, he isn't Anne. Why should Anne learn at Joe's speed? Anne isn't Joe. Each person learns in his own way. One person may learn hand levitation first, but that may be the last thing another person learns. Yet another might learn automatic writing before he learns anything else about a trance state. We have to be willing. I may discover that I can visualize more and more clearly certain things, and I ought to enjoy that particular thing I can visualize, never finding fault with the capacity of my unconscious to learn and to do things.

Dissociating Thinking and Doing

Establishing a Reverse Set to Disrupt Ordinary Consciousness and Induce Trance: "Is Your Name John Jones?"

The next topic that has been mentioned is this topic of trance deepening techniques. But there is another topic that I want to discuss as a preliminary, and that is this matter of inducing trances in various situations, and of discovering your own capacity to learn something about autohypnosis. If I were to ask Dr. Brody, "Is your name Joe Blow?", he would say, "No." He would probably resist the idea of telling me his name is Joe Blow. He wouldn't like the sound of that.

So often you will find your patient adhering steadfastly to his conscious understandings. I have used Dr. Brody and the name of Joe Blow to illustrate the possible ramifications of such understandings. But, you know, in going into a trance, in deepening a trance, in teaching a resistant subject to go into a trance, sometimes what you need to teach or to learn for yourself is the difference between thinking and doing.

Not long ago a patient came into my office and said, "I have had dozens of people try to hypnotize me, and I can't go into a trance. I just can't." I had the feeling the subject could go into a trance if he could get clarified in his own mind, so I began a series of questions.

"What is your name?" I asked.

"You know darned well what my name is," he responded. "I gave it to you, and you wrote it down on that sheet of paper. You not only wrote my name, you wrote my address. I don't know why you ask my name when you already know it."

"You know what do do now?" I said.

"Certainly," he answered.

"Do you know that I know it?" I asked.

"Yes," he said, "I know that you know it, and I can't see any sense in your asking me."

"Can I change your name?" I asked.

"No, you can't change my name," he answered. "I am the only person who can change my name, and then I would have to do it legally. I would have to go to court and petition for the change."

"So your name can't be changed?" I said. "All right, but tell me this. Tell me that your name is John Jones."

"My name is not John Jones," he retorted.

"I know that," I said. "But tell me that your name is John Jones."

"Well," he said, "I won't do that. My name isn't John Jones."

"Do I know that?" I asked.

"Certainly you do."

"Do you know it?"

"Certainly."

"All right," I continued, "tell me that your name is John Jones."

"IT IS NOT!" he answered emphatically.

I asked him how many times he had to explain to me that his name was not John Jones. Did he really believe that I knew it now? Could he tell me that his name was John Jones? It took quite a while for that man to understand that he could think, *My name is George Washington,* and nod his head yes; and when I asked, "Is your name John Jones?", he could nod his head yes while he was thinking, *It is George Washington.* The man needed to know the difference between neck muscle action and his thinking; he had to know definitely that his neck muscle action couldn't change his name.

Now I asked him, "I don't know your name, do I?" It was such a struggle for him to shake his head no, but after I had gotten him to answer a whole series of questions in which his head movement answers were contrary to his thinking answers then I could slip over into questions in which his head movement agreed with his thinking: "And you are not in a trance now, are you? But you want to go into a trance, don't you?" And so I would get a positive and a negative answer in accord with my questions and in accord with his understandings and his desires. "And you don't know that you are going into a trance, do you?"

> Eds: This is a double bind question. If the patient answers yes, he is acknowledging that he doesn't know he is going into trance. That is, he is going into trance without awareness of it. If the patient answers no, it literally means that he didn't know he was going into trance—which again implies that he is, in fact, going into trance.

He shook his head no. He didn't know that he was. That sort of question. I got him to divorce his thinking from his action, and thus his action was his response. As soon as I got him willing to divorce his thinking from his response, then I could start enlisting responses—positive or negative—as befitted the situation; and, sure enough, he went into a trance quite satisfactorily.[8]

Trance Deepening

Summating Simple and Limited Responses to Deepen Trance

Now this is an awfully important point for you to discover: that it isn't so important for you to insist to me that you are a man, or that you are a woman, or that you are standing up or that you are sitting down, or that you are lying down. You can think whatever you please, but also you are competent enough to respond. And so in the deepening of a trance your essential task is that of enlisting more and more responses from your patient.

Also bear in mind that it isn't the degree of significance that is important in the response. The response that is simple and limited can be utterly important, so long as you get a large number of them. So, for instance, instead of trying to compel the patient to relax his entire body, say rather, "I would like to have you feel relaxed in your little finger, and you can wiggle it just a little bit to show me that you are relaxed in the little finger." And then you get the patient's third finger relaxed, and the middle finger, and the index finger, and the thumb. You ask him to nod his head if he knows that this is Sunday afternoon, and he nods his head again, and he knows that he has nodded his head, and he nods it a third time. "And it was no real trouble to nod the head, was it?" And he shakes his head no. And so you build up one little response after another.

Trance Deepening via Arithmetic Progression

Yet another perspective that you want to create in your patient is an awareness of arithmetic progression. That is, if you say one penny this week, two pennies next week, four the following, eight the following, then sixteen, thirty-two, and so on—just doubling it fifty-two times—in a year's time there isn't that much money in the United States. One of my sons thought there might be a thousand dollars at the end of the year following my procedure. So I gave him the task of figuring it out arithmetically, and he discovered what a task that was. He couldn't possibly read the number. And so you ask your patient to get one ten-thousandth of a degree deeper into the trance. You build up the concept of doubling that amount, and then doubling it again, until the patient understands the concept of arithmetic progression. You are giving him a feeling that he is responding, even at an infinitesimal level, because as the trance deepening doubles again and again and again, it really deepens so very, very rapidly. The deepening technique is only the matter of eliciting more and more responses that are easier, and yet easier still, to carry out.

Trance Deepening via Hand Levitation

Utilizing Questions the Conscious Mind Cannot Answer to Facilitate Hand Levitation

Then there is the technique wherein you create for the patient a situation in which his unconscious can really function. For example, you ask the person if he understands what hand levitation is. Then you show him that the right hand can levitate upward, and the left hand can levitate upward. There is a slow, gradual, automatic movement, and he really doesn't know too much about hand levitation, but he can learn it. *And then you can ask him a question he can't answer consciously. There are a lot of questions that can't be answered consciously.* For example, the palm of your hand is here. Your conscious mind can think, *I would like to have the right hand lift up first;* or it can think, *I would like to have the left hand lift up.* But you don't know what the unconscious will choose. It may choose this hand, it may choose that hand; you don't know, it may choose both hands; it may choose to push downward. There are at least four possibilities: push down with the right and lift up with the left, or vice versa. You just don't know what the unconscious is going to do, and, therefore, you can ask your patient to look at his hands and see what the answer is so far as the unconscious mind is concerned. And as he looks at his hands and waits for his unconscious mind to decide if it will be the right, if it will be the left, it is his unconscious mind that has come forth; it is his unconscious mind that is in control; and it is his unconscious mind that is watching that hand, as well as his conscious mind.

You can then ask the question, "Are you in a trance?", and the patient can consciously reply, "Oh, no, I am not in a trance." And he can want to believe that so desperately that his conscious mind says, "No, I am not in a trance," but his unconscious mind is lifting his hand—and so he is in a trance without his knowledge.

Trance Without Awareness

Indirect Amnesia and the Forgotten Appointment

This is another point I think all of you professionals need to recognize, and a lot of your patients need to recognize; and that is the possibility of going into a trance without being aware of it. I will give you an example.

A patient came to me and said: "I have been a patient of yours for quite some time. I have asked you repeatedly to hypnotize me. You told me that I am not a suitable patient for hypnosis, that hypnosis is not a proper technique to use on me. But I want to be hypnotized, and I demand that you put me in a trance, and don't give me any more argument. I want you to hypnotize me. Now, get going on it." And he straightened up in his chair, folded his arms across his chest, and sat there literally daring me.

"All right," I said, "I would like to have you relax all over, very quiet and at ease, and slowly begin to get tired and sleepy."

"Not that kind of suggestion," he said, "be emphatic and really put forth some effort."

And I kept right on, "And slowly, gently your eyelids will close, and you will go more and more asleep."

"Now listen," he demanded. "I want some genuine suggestions. Be forceful and compelling and demanding!"

But even as he gave me my orders, I kept right on. "And slowly get more and more tired, and more and more sleepy."

He kept on heckling me and demanding that I do a decent job, and ten minutes to the hour I looked at the clock, and he said: "You have wasted another one of my hours that I have to pay you for, and you didn't put me in a trance. I remember the session from beginning to end. I have been sitting here all that time listening to the weak, ineffectual, incompetent way in which you have tried to put me in a trance—talking to me as if I were some old lady that needed to be soothed. I can remember, verbatim, every ineffectual thing that you said!"

"Yes," I agreed. "You can remeber every thing that I said. You were sitting less than six feet away. *You are here in the office, and you can remember what I said in the office.* You were here and you can remember."

> Eds: Both parts of this compound suggestion are obviously true. Thus the patient's conscious mind accepts the suggestion in its entirety without recognizing the hidden implications. The first clause, "You are here in the office," implies a limitation on the second half, "you do remember every word I said." The remembering is actually limited to

60

"You are here in the office." This form of implication illustrates a special case of the more general forms of indirect suggestion explicated elsewhere.[9]

He retorted, "The next time I come here I want you to put me in a trance and I want proof."

"The next time you come," I said, "I'll have proof."

"Well," he snapped, "you haven't got it now! I remember every word you said."

"Yes," I agreed. *"You are here in the office, and you do remember every word I said."* So I gave him an appointment for the following Wednesday.

On Wednesday I met him out in the waiting room. He came in, looked at me rather peculiarly, asking, "Did I keep last Monday's appointment?"

"Why do you ask?" I said. "If you had kept the appointment certainly you would know it."

"I can't remember whether I kept it or not."

"What do you remember?" I asked.

"I remember that I was sitting in my car," he began, "and I couldn't remember whether I had just come back from seeing you, or whether I was just getting in the car to drive to your office. I looked at my watch—it was half past six—and I knew it was too late, so I figured I had broken the appointment. But I know I have to pay you for it anyway."

"Let's go in the office," I said.

As soon as he had crossed over the threshold into the office, he said: "I did too keep my appointment! I was here, and you tried to hypnotize me, and I can remember everything you said, and you tried so weakly."

"Yes, that is right," I said. "By the way, there is a magazine out in the waiting room I want to discuss with you. Let's go out and get it."

We went out to the waiting room and he said, "Did I keep my Monday appointment?", so we went back round that question again. Then we went back into the office and he remembered that he had kept the appointment. The third time back in the

61

office he said: "This is the third time. Why can't I remember out in the other room?"

"Let's go out to the other room," I suggested. But he couldn't remember out in the other room. And then we went back into the office where, of course, he could remember everything. I pointed out the situation to him, and that ended his demands, because now he knew.

You need to know that some of your patients will react that way, and don't think that you have failed because they have their own goals. You must develop your own willingness to believe in yourselves, and to expect your patients to accomplish certain things. Now I was willing to let that patient heckle me. I allowed him to sneak into a deep trance without his awareness of that fact, and I was willing to let him go into a deep trance in his own particular way: In the office he could remember everything about the session we had had, but out in the waiting room (and elsewhere) he could have a complete amnesia for that session.

You must be willing to let the patient have his recollection in your office and his amnesia outside of your office; you must be willing to let him experience certain phenomena in your office and certain phenomena outside of your office; you must be willing to let him have one type of experience now and another type of experience later to signify the difference between success and failure in your use of hypnosis. *I had that willingness to let the patient have no amnesia in my office but an implied amnesia everywhere else.* His achievement of that partial amnesia served tremendously to alter his total behavior. He had his absolute proof at the time he asked for it, and he was willing to receive that proof.[10]

Group Hypnosis

Autohypnotic Techniques Structuring a Self/Other Rapport to Include All Contingencies

Let's move on to the matter of teaching autohypnosis in a group situation. Since we have a group right here, it is perfectly possible for all of you to take a lesson in group hypnosis right now. Actually, some of you have taken advantage of my lecture this afternoon—just as you took advantage of it this morning—to go into a trance. You went into the trance this morning and this afternoon, not by virtue of my effort to put you in a trance, but by virtue of your own interest in going into a trance. And so you merely took advantage of my presence here; you took advantage of my speaking as a central point of orientation whereby you could distract your conscious mind and allow your unconscious mind the opportunity of going into a trance. And every one of you that went into a trance, went into both the autohypnotic trance and the heterohypnotic trance, and you did it in this way: you went into the trance in rapport, primarily, with yourselves.

Now all of you know in your own unconscious minds that in going into a trance in an audience situation you reserve for yourself the right to rouse up any time you please, and you reserve the right to go back into the trance any time you please. In other words, you establish rapport with yourselves and you exercise that rapport with yourselves, but you also are kind enough to include me in the rapport.

In autohypnosis you can go into the trance in rapport only with yourself, or, if you wish, you can go into the trance in rapport also with X and with Y and with Z; you can even arrange it so that you are in rapport with that person who comes to your door and rings the bell quite unexpectedly—a person who has no particular part in your total trance situation; you can go into the autohypnotic trance in rapport with the telephone so that an adequate response can be made to all possible contingencies.

Let's summarize. In this matter of going into an autohypnotic trance your first orientation should be to your situation: that you want to go into the trance; that you do not want to handicap yourself in any way; that you can rely upon your unconscious mind to answer the doorbell or the telephone or to speak to anybody who walks into your office. In short, you can meet any contingency, likely or unlikely, that might arise. Once you think that through—that you can meet any contingency, likely or unlikely—you can go into an autohypnotic trance and you can handle things as effectively as if you were in the ordinary waking state. Thus, you can send a good autohypnotic subject downtown into the thickest of traffic jams, and he can drive with absolute safety once he understands that he can meet any contingency. In fact, he can probably drive a lot more safely because he will have his mind on the driving, and he won't be wool-gathering the way so many of us do when we are carrying out a habitual activity.

Utilizing Autohypnosis

Pivotal Role of Expectancy in Hypnotic Learning: The 25-Cent Student Experiment

Now I notice that a number of you are interested in autohypnosis and in utilizing this situation. I also notice that many of you definitely are not interested in openly utilizing it, while some of you are utilizing it but are unaware of that fact. You are totally unaware of your facial rigidity, of your eyeball rigidity, of your failure to make associated movements, of your failure to adjust to any of the disturbances around you.[11]

For all of you who have achieved your autohypnotic learning, I would like to have you continue that learning. I would like to have you aware of the fact that you can utilize what you have learned today over and over again throughout the coming year, and that you can develop that learning in any particular direction that you wish to develop it. You see, there is a need for you to appreciate the fact that you are competent. I do not know how well you understand the role of attitudes of expectancy, attitudes of willingness [in the outcome of your endeavors], but I can think of one psychological experiment that has been done repeatedly to illustrate.

You take 100 students and divide them into two groups—Group A and Group B. Then you take another student and make him your impartial assistant. You keep this assistant isolated in a room while you explain to Group A: "There are two groups of students here, the A group and the B group. I am going to send each of you in Group A into a room, one at a time, with one member of the B group. You are not to talk to one another; you are just to walk casually around the room. After about two minutes a third person will enter the room. He will not speak. You just continue to wander around casually, and then after a couple of minutes he will walk up to you and he will hand you a 25-cent piece."

Then you explain the same thing to Group B except that you state that, "after about two minutes, the third person will walk up to you and he will hand you a dollar bill."

To the student who is assisting you, you explain: "You are to go into this room over and over again. Each time, you will find two different students there. You will look them over casually, walk around the room casually, never saying a word. After a couple of minutes you will walk up to one and give him a quarter; you will walk up to the other and give him a dollar bill." In other words, the student assistant has absolutely no clues.

In about eighty percent of the trials, Group A members got the quarter and Group B members got the dollar. Why?—because Group A had a 25-cent expectancy and Group B had a dollar expectancy. The one group had a larger relative expectancy than the other, and the student didn't know which to give the quarter to and which to give the dollar to. But he responded to the minimal cue of the larger expectancy, and he didn't even realize that that was what was happening. So you have a nice, controlled experiment.

When you bear in mind how thoroughly the attitude of expectancy can record itself in such a concrete way, then you also had better bear in mind that your own attitude of expectancy toward yourself can yield the same results. That is why you ought to be able to expect yourself to do automatic writing. Surely you know how to write. Surely you have put on the brake when you have been riding in the back seat of a car; surely you have tensed your mouth and your throat and your vocal cords while listening to a stutterer trying to say a word; surely you have opened your mouth so widely that it was painful when you tried to feed that baby that wouldn't open its mouth. You know all of those things; therefore, you can really expect yourself to do automatic writing.

Inducing Blindness to Facilitate Audition

Utilizing Sensory Interassociations and Interdependencies for Hypnotic Learning

When it comes to this matter of visualization, however, you must remember that some people possess the ability to visualize while others do not. Some people can visualize in that sensory modality but cannot visualize in the auditory modality. Some people can hallucinate sounds but not visions, while others can see things but cannot hallucinate sounds. And still others find it difficult to develop a sense of numbness.

Now there is another aspect to this issue that I want you to bear in mind. This morning I mentioned the use of hyperasthesia to induce anesthesia. I want you to bear in mind that just as the toe bone is connected to the foot bone, and the foot bone is connected to the anklebone, so it is in many a person's psychological functioning. Thus, visualization capabilities are connected to abilities to form auditory images, and sometimes the ability to visualize is connected in another way with the sense of hearing. All of you have had the experience where you will sit down and listen to a radio program of an orchestra, and you close your eyes and turn your best ear toward the radio—trying to pick out the woodwinds or the brass or the number of violins—because you exclude vision from your listening. And so sometimes you might bring about a visual blindness or a closing of the eyes in order to produce better auditory hallucinations; sometimes you enable a person to become hypnotically deaf by virtue of the fact that you have intensified his ability to visualize.

You ought to keep in mind this interrelationship between the various modalities of behavior. That is why I urge all of you to work with each other, and with normal college students, so that you can experiment with the various types of behavior. And the more you learn about the interdependencies and the interassociations of various types of behavior, the better knowledge you will have of hypnosis and of its use.

DEMONSTRATION

Now I am going to offer some demonstrations of trance induction, and I am going to call upon various members of the audience.

Easing into Trance

Utilizing Response Attentiveness, Not Knowing, and Ideodynamic Comfort, Relaxation, and Well-Being to Induce Trance; Ultradian Cycle, Parasympathetic, and Right-Hemispheric Response Readiness for Trance

Erickson (E): Now tell me, Paul, did you go into a trance today?

Paul (P): *I don't know.*

E: You don't know if you went into a trance. What is your guess? What is your opinion.

P: I was very *relaxed*.

E: You were very relaxed. Anything else?

P: No.

E: What do you mean by relaxed?

P: *Very comfortable.*

E: Very comfortable.

P: *A sense of well-being. I felt very comfortable.*

Eds: While this may appear to be a bit of casual, introductory small-talk about "comfort," "relaxation," and "well-being," much more is actually involved. As Erickson reveals in his closing summary of the demonstration, he had carefully selected this subject from the audience because he was already manifesting the relaxed behavior characteristic of "response attentiveness" and the "common everyday trance." That is, Paul had already drifted into an altered state as he listened to Erickson discuss hypnosis.

This involves the ideodynamic principle of trance induction: simply hearing a discussion about hypnosis, dissociation, and altered states tends to evoke personal associations and memories of the altered states we have all experienced in the ordinary course of everyday life. These associations and memories tend in turn to evoke the actual experience of trance behavior in the here-and-now. This is particularly likely to occur if we happen to be in that period of our ultradian cycle when parasympathetic and right-hemispheric tendencies are most manifest. A subjective sense of "comfort," "relaxation," and—if our attitudes permit it—"a sense of well-being," are all highly characteristic of this phase of the ultradian cycle.

When Paul responds to Erickson's first question with the response, "I don't know," Paul is unwittingly validating his already altered state. A sense of *not knowing* implies that left-hemispheric functioning is in abeyance: this, of course, is exactly what one would expect when in the ultradian period of relaxation (right-hemispheric dominance).

Resistance to Trance

Converting Unconscious Defense into Conscious Cooperation and Utilizing Resistance to Build Rapport: Minimal Cues of Behavioral Agitation

E: How do you feel right now?

P: Not too comfortable.

E: How do you know *you don't feel too comfortable right now?*

P: Everybody is staring at me.

E: Did you announce to the audience that *you were uncomfortable?*

P: When?

E: When you first sat down.

P: No.

E: You didn't. Are you doing anything that tells the audience that *you are uncomfortable right now?* That is right. You looked right at it, didn't you. You were playing with the ring on your finger in an agitated way, weren't you?

P: That's right.

E: In an agitated way, and *I am deliberately making you uncomfortable in an agitated way.* Isn't that right? Do you mind?

P: No.

E: *But you do mind, don't you?*

P: *I don't think so.*

E: *Could you think that way—that you do mind?*

P: *Yes, I could.*

E: Yes, you could mind. But *you'd rather not be uncomfortable,* isn't that right? Are you beginning to recall some of the feelings you had earlier today?

P: A little bit.

E: How much have you used hypnosis?

P: Not very much.

E: Are you a dentist?

P: Yes.

> Eds: Relaxed as the subject initially appeared to be, Erickson nonetheless notes some agitation minimally manifest in Paul's absentminded playing with his ring. This agitation could interfere with the forthcoming hypnotic work, so Erickson undertakes an appropriate way of managing it. The first step in this appropriate management is to acknowledge the truth that Erickson is the source of Paul's agitation. When Paul responds, "I don't think so," to Erickson's question about whether he minds being agitated, Paul is betraying the dissociated state he is experiencing: on an ideomotor level he is manifesting agitation by playing with his ring while in front of a large audience; on a verbal level, however, he cannot acknowledge that he "minds" experiencing this sense of agitation. Erickson then makes a minimal effort to bridge the dissociation between Paul's motor and verbal levels by asking, *"Could you think that way—that you do mind?"* Erickson has done

a bit of healing with this question, as Paul responds, "Yes, I could."

He then allows the dissociation to return for hypnotic purposes when he continues with, *"But you'd rather not be uncomfortable, isn't that right?"* What was originally an unconscious dissociation mediated by automatic mechanisms of defense has now been converted into a conscious choice of dissociation. This facilitates the hypnotic process by allowing the subject to cooperate comfortably with Erickson, even while in the unaccustomed glare of a large audience.

While Erickson has managed to help convert Paul's unconscious resistance into a conscious choice to cooperate, we must note that he has not manipulated Paul into doing something he does not want to do. Rather, he has helped all parts of Paul to cooperate together for a more rewarding life experience. Erickson did not believe hypnosis could be used to manipulate people into doing anything they did not want to do, and he believed he had provided adequate experimental proof of this.[12]

This short interaction thus illustrates Erickson's facile genius in dealing with resistance and defense. A less acute hypnotherapist might simply have congratulated himself on recognizing Paul's readiness to be a cooperative subject, and then proceeded hypnotically with some modicum of success. Erickson, however, also noted the minimal resistance and took care to discharge and/or utilize it as the first step in facilitating an even more adequate rapport. That rapport could then provide the basis of an even more profound hypnotic experience later on.

Hand Levitation

Double-Binding Questions, Contingent Suggestions, and "Not Knowing"

E: All right. Will you place your hands on your thighs, feet flat on the floor, and now look at your hands. *Which one is going to lift first?* **Do you know?**

P: I don't know.

E: You really don't know. Lifting, lifting. Only your unconscious knows. **You are going to start lifting, lifting, and** *will your hand lift before your eyes close?* **You really don't know, and your eyes have been closed before your hands came to rest—relaxing, relaxing, lifting up, lifting. That is right. Take a deep breath, and one of those hands continues to lift. Lifting, lifting, lifting.** *And then as your eyelids close your hand will lift.* **And I am going to talk about you to the audience.**

> Eds: Erickson uses a pair of double binding questions in this hand levitation induction. When he asks, "Which one is going to lift first?", he is introducing a double bind: trance will become manifest, whichever hand lifts. He also immediately distracts Paul's attention with the question, "Do you know?" *When Paul responds with "I don't know," this indicates that his conscious mind has relinquished the task of deciding which hand is going to lift: he is now leaving it up to his unconscious.*
>
> Erickson then introduces another double bind question: "Will your hand lift before your eyes close?" This question focuses on possibilities while allowing Paul's own system the freedom to decide. The question is nonetheless a double bind because, again, trance will be facilitated whichever possibility is chosen. Apparently Paul's eyelids began closing first, so Erickson utilized this question to facilitate the hand levitation. He then followed it up with the *contingent suggestion,* "And then as your eyelids close, your hand will lift."

Indirect Posthypnotic Suggestion

Minimal Cues of Trance Readiness and Resistance; Subtle Posthypnotic Suggestion for Autohypnotic Learning.

E: [To audience] Now, I had this gentleman come up to the front because *he was an excellent hypnotic subject.* He really fixed his gaze on me, and he remained unaware of the people beside him so that even when they moved in such a way that should have attracted his attention, he did not notice. And he kept on looking at me, and he got awfully self-conscious when I raised the question of autohypnosis. So I had the feeling that he would come up and show a great deal of agitation and resistance—and he did an awfully nice job. He made it awfully clear. And then when I suggested the raising of his hands I offered the alternative of the closing of his eyes. You saw the overly dramatic drawing of a breath, and then you saw the movement of his scalp, the movement of his eyebrows, the blinking of his eyes as he started to close them, and then the increased swallowing reflex—because he is resistant in this situation. And I very deliberately emphasized the fact that he was self-conscious, and I made him more self-conscious, because it seemed to him to be an intolerable situation. What can he do about the situation? He is a professionally trained man, this is a professional group; he knows there is no malice or vindictiveness involved; he knows that it is a teaching situation out of which his own unconscious is going to organize a wealth of understandings. And so, because of the nice way in which he attended, and the fact that he did develop a good autohypnotic trance while sitting at the table, I thought I would single him out. *As a teaching subject he shows some resistance, but he will undoubtedly do more of his learning by himself tomorrow, or next week, or the following week, rather than here in this situation.*

> Eds: In this intellectual explanation to the audience, Erickson is actually reinforcing the subject indirectly with remarks such as, "He was an excellent hypnotic subject." The final sentence of this purported talk to the audience is actually an indirect posthypnotic suggestion to Paul for further autohypnotic learning. The first portion of this sentence, "As a teaching subject he shows some resistance," is a truth the subject can accept. This acceptance tends to open a yes set for him then to accept the second portion of the sentence, "he will undoubtedly do more of his learning by himself tomorrow, or next week, or the following week"—which is the indirect posthypnotic suggestion.[13]

Involuntary Ideomotor Movements

Head Nodding and Smiling Indicating Patient's Self-Discovery of Trance

You see, I have talked about him freely to you, and in spite of the fact that I have said things to intensify his self-consciousness, notice instead that his facial muscles are beginning to iron out, and that there is a tendency for him to go into a trance. His breathing has become more regular, and there is a greater ease about him, and I wonder if you can see it. And shortly, *when I say there is a greater ease about him, he will nod or shake his head* slowly, gradually to signify. Now, notice that he smiles at that—at the shaking of his own head—and you know why. And now he can nod his head or shake his head if he agrees or disagrees with me. The nodding of the head is involuntary, and it took him a little by surprise.

E: Is that why you smiled?

P: [Nods his head yes.]

That is right. And I emphasize this because all of you need to know that the sudden smile, the apparent resistances, are a recognition on the part of this subject that he, himself, is going into a trance. And that particular smile at that particular moment was his discovery that the nodding of his head was in part involuntary—that he, literally, had had nothing to do with it.

P: [Apparently, he both nods and shakes his head.]

E: Yes it is, and no it isn't, and that is so correct.

Time distortion as an issue really isn't important to him in this situation, but it is important to him as a professional man to understand something about it. And it is really quite important, and so the right answer, the correct answer, was the one which actually left him much more confused—but that is all right.

Understanding Response Delay

Time Distortion and Ideomotor Signaling as Trance Indicators

This calls to my attention another matter. You must have a willingness to wait, to not get agitated or excited or disturbed because things don't happen at the moment you suggest that they happen.

E: And the hand is lifting higher and higher. It is the right hand, and it is lifting, lifting higher. I would like to have you enjoy it, especially when you feel the elbow bending. Now with the lifting of the hand you ought to bear in mind that you need to let the elbow bend.

Now this delayed response is often something that you can treasure because it tells you that your patient is going to learn, and it tells you the importance of the patient recognizing his own time, his own speed of learning. And just because you suggested the lifting of his hand doesn't mean he is going to follow your suggestion immediately.

Now as I observe him I can see that he is experiencing considerable time distortion, because I don't believe he knows how long that delay was. But I don't think it is important to him, and I am going to ask him to answer the question, and he can answer it positively or negatively by nodding his head or shaking his head.

E: Is it really important to you whether or not you know the length of time?

Three-Stage Hypnotic Suggestion

Not Knowing, Questions, and Expectancy to Facilitate and Quicken Hypnotic Responses

[Erickson apparently brings a second subject onto the stage and proceeds to work with both subjects alternately.]

E: And just keep sleeping deeper and deeper all the time. And keep sleeping deeper and deeper, Joe. And of course you are curious. *You really don't know; you don't know whether you are in a trance or not,* and some of the time you keep your eyes open, and some of the time you keep your eyes closed, and *you are uncertain about the whole thing.*

[Shifting subjects] And Paul, keep right on sleeping, and *I am going to ask your left hand to start lifting [pause], and now your left hand will start lifting.*

We already know that Paul takes his time. We've had that demonstrated, and so I told him, "I am going to ask your left hand to lift." ... First I said I *was going to ask* his left hand to lift, which didn't mean he should lift it. Then I said, "And now your left hand *will start lifting,*" to which he could make a much more immediate response.

And how do you teach your patients who tend to be slow to respond more quickly? This is the technique that you employ: *you raise the question of what they can do, you tell them you are going to expect them to do it, and then you tell them to do it.* You get a much quicker response that way.

E: And now, Paul, your right hand could go down.

And you see how much more quickly his right hand started down? Almost immediately. And so I am teaching him how to respond much more quickly.

Posthypnotic Suggestion

Utilizing Inevitabilities as Associative Cues

E: And your right hand can go higher and higher, and enjoy it—really enjoy it. And don't let my speaking interrupt it. Just thoroughly enjoy it. [Pause] All right, Paul, do you feel that you have had enough experience so that you'll be willing to keep on learning thoroughly after you sit down? Feel comfortable about it now, Paul. And do you feel that you know how to follow out posthypnotic suggestion? And would next Friday be a nice time to review this—being up here on the platform? Would next Friday be a nice time to review it? All right. We will agree on that. And now, to get back to your seat, will you rouse up just enough to get back to your seat and sit down?

> Eds: Note that Erickson is careful to tie his posthypnotic suggestion to a definite time in the future that is an inevitability. It is inevitable that Friday will come, and when Friday comes it will serve as an associative cue for Paul to receive this posthypnotic suggestion.

Confusion and Not Knowing in Trance

E: [Shifting subjects] All right, Joe, you can also *rouse up and review your learnings back at your seat.*

J: Do you want me to go back to my seat?

E: May I repeat what you said to the audience?: "Do you want me to go back to my seat" was his question. Now, I haven't answered you, have I, Joe?

J: *I am confused.*

E: You are confused. I wonder why. You are doing it all right. You are doing it very nicely. I don't think we could have had a better demonstration. Why did you raise that question, Joe?

J: *I don't know.*

E: You don't know. And you really don't know, do you? By the way, did you know that Paul was up here? Where is he?

J: He went back to his seat.

E: Why?

J: You told him.

E: I told him. I think all of you recognize the failure of follow-through in thinking.

> Eds: Erickson's initial statement that Joe can rouse up and review his learnings back at his seat contains the implication that he must go back to his seat. But Joe responds with confusion and not knowing. Why? It could be that Joe is still being influenced by Erickson's earlier suggestions [two sections back] to the effect of, "You really don't know; you don't know whether you are in a trance or not ... You are uncertain about the whole thing." These suggestions of not knowing and uncertainty may still be active within Joe so that he is not able to grasp Erickson's implication that he can return to his seat. Erickson describes this as a "failure of follow-through in thinking."

Techniques for Facilitating Hypnotic Amnesia

Expectation Versus Direct Suggestion; Ratifying Subjects'
Trance Experiences

One of the questions listed here for me to discuss is how to induce an amnesia. Usually you don't have to induce it; you just let your subject show the amnesia. Too often practitioners try to induce an AMNESIA, thereby naming, tagging, emphasizing that "this is what I want you to forget"; instead, you induce your amnesia by your expectations for it.

E: By the way, Joe, do you think you could develop hypnotic amnesia?

J: I don't know.

E: That is right. You don't really know. That is all right. Do you remember that Paul was told to go back to his seat? Now, what are you thinking of?

J: Nothing.

And all the rest of you know what you are thinking, but Joe does have an amnesia. And he is doing very, very nicely with that amnesia, and I am able to talk about it and I am able to scurry around it, and he still has his amnesia. Now, you may think that I am over-emphasizing this point, but I assure you that you need to know what words mean, and you need to know how you approach ideas. Every one of you can appreciate the need for scientific accuracy in your professional work. In some aspects of your work it is tremendously important not to be a fraction of a millimeter too far away or too close. In the matter of dealing with human nature, human psychology, human futures, you need to have an accuracy in the words you use as tools, and so the more you learn about the effectiveness of words the better off you are.

E: What are you thinking about, Paul?

P: I don't know.

E: You were daydreaming, to the best of your knowledge, isn't that right?

P: Yes, but I can't remember about what.

E: You can't remember about what. That is right, for when it began you had gone into a trance. Weren't you up here, Paul?

P: Yes.

E: Why did you leave? [Pause] Yes, why did you leave? I asked you to. *And that you can remember.*

P: Yes, I can remember that.

E: That *you can remember.*

What have I told him really? The implication of what I said was that he could remember, and his reply was: "Yes, I can remember that." His unconscious replied for him, because Paul is going to have some amnesias, too. I am risking damaging those amnesias by calling his attention to them. Joe, however, is in a situation where I can talk freely because he is still here in this chair. That is where he went into a trance.

Therapeutic Trance

Receptivity, Response Attentiveness, and Catalepsy; Training in Negative Hallucination and Total Body Anesthesia

E: Did you know you went into a trance, Joe?

J: I'm not sure.

E: You're not sure. Are you right-handed or left-handed?

J: Right-handed.

E: You are not sure, though, [that you were in a trance]? How could you find out? Do you know any way to find out?

J: I know I had the levitation. That was an indication.

E: It was an indication. What else?

J: *I felt different.*

E: You felt different. Anything else?

J: *I wasn't conscious that I was sitting in front of the group here. It didn't make any difference.*

E: Did you pretty much forget about the group? *How much did you forget the group?*

J: *Completely.*

E: You forgot about the group when your eyes were open. Is that right?

J: Yes.

E: Maybe you were in a trance. That is right. Maybe you are in a trance right now, and don't know it.

I think all of you can recognize that Joe is in a trance. There is a certain rigidity and unresponsiveness about him. He isn't in the kind of trance you would usually employ for major surgery, but I think you could do quite a number of minor things with him in the way of surgery. I think you could do quite a bit with him as far as dentistry is concerned. You could do a great deal with him psychotherapeutically, because he is going to listen to what the therapist says. He is going to hear it; he is going to understand it; he is going to apply it; he is not going to be attentive to any of the distracting influences around him. This is the type of trance that I like to use extensively, and I think all of you can appreciate the fact that he is in a trance. And it is a trance that you don't use for testing or for irrelevant purposes. *Catalepsy is present, and slowly, gradually, Joe is going to discover that he can maintain an absolute negative hallucination for everything around him at the visual level, at the auditory level; and sooner or later he can develop a complete anesthesia of his body.*

> Eds: Again under the guise of giving the audience an intellectual explanation, Erickson is actually giving Joe casual, indirect suggestions for learning to maintain absolute negative hallucinations and anesthesia. Joe indicated that he

81

was ready to experience a negative hallucination when he said, "I wasn't conscious that I was sitting in front of the group here." He indicated that he might be ready to experience a complete body anesthesia when he offered, "I felt different" in trance. This is therefore an unusually clear illustration of how Erickson would recognize the minimal manifestations of spontaneous hypnotic phenomena and then seek to maximize them.

Trance Termination

Catalepsy as a Segmentation Phenomenon

E: *Now, Joe, sooner or later you will want to learn something about posthypnotic suggestion; and you really want to learn something about posthypnotic suggestion.* But first there is something that you need to learn a great deal more about, and that is the spasticity of the deltoid muscles—spasticity of your shoulder muscles; and *I would like to have you willing to feel the spasticity of your shoulder muscles even after you are awake.* Do you understand, Joe? That is right. Now close your eyes, take a deep breath, and *slowly awaken comfortably, except for the right shoulder. Wake up, Joe.* Are you awake? Do you want to go back to your seat now? Will you, please!

> Eds: Erickson ends this phase of his work with Joe with the time binding posthypnotic suggestion, "Sooner or later you will want to learn something about posthypnotic suggestion." This is a preparation for the more direct suggestion that immediately follows, "And you really want to learn something about posthypnotic suggestion." This, in turn, is a preparation for the surprising, specific suggestion, "I would like to have you willing to feel the spasticity of your shoulder muscle even after you are awake." Why? We can only speculate that Erickson noticed that Joe had some sort of involuntary spasticity in his shoulder that he was not aware of. Having Joe become aware of it after he awakens may be the first step to resolving it.

Erickson then ends with, "Slowly awaken comfortably, except for that right shoulder. Wake up, Joe." Erickson appears to be making use of what he sometimes called the "segmented trance": all the body awakens except for one part which remains in trance for therapeutic purposes. Joe's shoulder would remain in a form of "catalepsy as a segmentation phenomenon."[14] Although Erickson appears to be abruptly ending his work with Joe at this point, we can assume he followed up and completed this therapeutic effort at a later time which was not recorded.

A Subtle Double Bind to be "Thoroughly Uncooperative"

E: [Erickson now addresses another member of the audience.] Now Bernice, will you come here? Tell me, Bernice, *will you be a thoroughly uncooperative patient?*

B: Uncooperative?

E: That is right. What are you thinking about?

B: I am waiting.

E: Never mind that. You're supposed to be uncooperative.

B: Shall I think uncooperatively?

E: [To audience] She wants to know if she should think uncooperatively. [To subject] You shoved up the sleeve on the left arm, didn't you—as if *you were girding for battle*. Isn't that right? What about your right sleeve. How about rolling that up, too?

B: It is already rolled up.

E: Is it rolled enough?

B: Do you want me to roll it up more?

E: You are weakening too fast.

B: Maybe I should close my eyes.

E: Why? More resistant if you close your eyes? Well, *why don't you close them.*

And she raised the question of closing her eyes, but she didn't do it, so I said, "Why don't you?" Didn't I take hold of the management of that situation in a simple way? *I'd like to have her uncooperative.*

> Eds: Although Erickson does not label it as such, he is here drawing attention to how he took "hold of the management of that situation in a simple way" with a subtle double bind. By telling Bernice to be uncooperative he is actually in control of her behavior: when Bernice acts uncooperatively at Erickson's bidding, she is actually cooperating with him. She is cooperating with him even though acting as if she is not. Thus she is in a double bind. Erickson continues with further double binding suggestions in the next section.

Utilizing Resistance in Hypnotic Induction

Prescribing the Symptom: Paradoxical or Reverse Suggestion and Surprising Questions

E: *Don't give me the opportunity of taking charge.* You could smile. That's it, wiggle your shoulders and *do your level best not to sit still.* That is right, *do your level best not to sit still.* You want to sit still. Well, of course, that is what I need to have you do. And you know that, and *are you gripping hard enough with your right or left hand?*

B: I will if you want me to.

E: **You will if I want you to.**

And I raised the question, "Are you gripping hard enough with your right or your left hand?" Now what am I doing here? I am compelling the subject to examine her right hand, examine her left hand, and I am compelling her. You see, one of the issues on this list for me to discuss is the question of how to use a patient's resistance. The answer is, you never try to overcome it—you try to use it.

> Eds: Erickson is using a form of paradoxical or reverse suggestion when *prescribes the symptom* to gain control over it when he says, "Don't give me the opportunity of taking charge... Do your level best not to sit still." Evidently he had noticed that the subject was restless or shifting about in her seat—perhaps as a manifestation of resistance. He utilizes this manifestation of resistance by suggesting that she continue it—thus making her resistance of manifestation of following his suggestions rather than resisting against them. He then further focuses her attention by asking, "Are you gripping hard enough with your right or left hand?" This peculiar question is probably surprising enough to depotentiate whatever other conscious preoccupation she might have had, and to initiate an inner search of her sensory experience to determine which hand is gripping hard enough. Thus the first three stages of the microdynamics of trance induction[15] have occurred, and the interaction is concluded with the subject's statement, "I will if you want me to." This clearly indicates that she is now following Erickson in a cooperative manner.

Ideomotor Movements in Trance Induction

Contingent Suggestions and Questions for Hand Levitation;
The Role of Confusion in Catalepsy

B: **You know, my heart is beating pretty fast. You will have to settle me down.**

E: I will have to settle you down a little bit. How much do you want your heart slowed down?

B: A reasonable rate.

E: A reasonable rate. Reasonable for this situation.

B: Real slow.

E: Not too slow, but the right amount in accord with this situation and in accord with the task you have to do. And *as your right hand lifts, will your heart slow down a bit?* Let us find out as it slowly lifts.

B: *I'm not at that stage yet.*

E: You are not at that stage yet. [To audience] There she has offered the promise—not at that stage *yet*—that implies she is going to be at that stage at some point.

B: I want to.

E: You want to. That is right. And slowly your hand comes up, and *I will take hold of the wrist.*

B: *Shall I raise it?*

E: That is right.

B: Because I want you to—

E: Because you want me to tell you.

And she raised the question of should she raise her hand voluntarily. And now the question has come up of, do I want her to hold her hand there voluntarily? Now I can discuss that question; I can raise the pros and cons and argue this way and argue that way—and yet never actually answer the question. And all the time I am talking about it, *her hand remains up there because she can't settle* that.

> Eds: When Erickson says, "I will take hold of the wrist," he is actually guiding her hand upward with a variety of subtle guiding touches.[16] Because subjects usually are not able to recognize Erickson's tactile cues as the reason for their arm movement, they frequently experience it as autonomous or involuntary. This involuntary aspect of their own body movement is inexplicable to them, and because of the context of the hypnotic situation they take it as evidence of having entered an altered or hypnotic state. In this case, however, the subject is confused by Erickson and asks, "Shall I raise it?" In his commentary to the audience he says, "her hand remains up there because she can't settle that," indicating his belief that the phenomenon of catalepsy is mediated at least in part by confusion ("because she can't settle *that*" [all the complex issues and subtle cues that she is receiving]).

The "Resistance Trance"

The Law of Reversed Effects; Anxiety Responses, Ideomotor Head Movements, and Hand Catalepsy as Ratifications of Trance

B: I'm just not getting into it.

E: You are just not getting into it enough, but you are doing very, very nicely. You came up here oriented primarily to go into a trance, Bernice, and I am using you to illustrate resistance and the utilization of that resistance. And you will either nod or shake your head in reply: In order to illustrate my points you have developed a different type of trance. Is that correct?

B: No...I don't know. I want you to put me in a trance.

E: Yes, you want me to put you in a kind of a trance that you are familiar with. Isn't that right?

B: I just want to know what it feels like.

E: You want to know what it feels like. Do you think you are in a trance right now?

B: I am afraid not.

E: You are afraid not. Now, I am going to touch you on the head.

B: I still feel my heart is beating too fast.

E: You still feel your heart is beating too fast.

B: I want to slow that heart down.

E: You want to slow that heart down.

B: My circulation is too fast.

E: Your circulation is too fast. And what else?

B: I may go to sleep if I have to calm down.

E: Will you go to sleep if you have to calm down? Maybe you are trying too hard. Now, are you in a trance? Let your head nod yes or no.

B: This way?

E: *Wait and see which way it nods*. Are you in a trance? Now wait and see. You didn't wait and see. You wait and see. Are you in a trance? Wait and see if your head nods yes. Have you ever realized how quickly the unconscious can do things and how it can slip things in. Your head nodded yes then, didn't it? Yes it did. Essentially you are in a trance. You have been in a trance right along.

B: Have I?

E: You didn't know it, but I wanted you to show resistances; I wanted you to illustrate the type of trance that these doctors ought to know about wherein the patient can swear, "I am not in a trance"; wherein the patient can argue and dispute and yet maintain a catalepsy that is just enough of a catalepsy to be convincing to the self. So often in psychotherapy patients need to do this sort of thing; so often in obstetrics patients need to do this sort of thing, so that the abdomen and the pelvis is free to go into a trance state. This element of dissociation in human behavior is very, very significant.

B: *I can't put my hand down.*

E: Well, why can't you put your hand down?

B: *It doesn't seem very natural.*

> Eds: Thus without her conscious mind understanding how or why, Bernice's unconscious carried out Erickson's original directive to "be a thoroughly uncooperative patient" by making her heart beat too fast. This was apparently the opposite of Bernice's conscious understanding of what trance behavior was like. This hyperactive type of behavior frequently is seized upon by the patient's conscious mind as proof of not being in trance. It is typically (and erroneously) believed that trance behavior is always tranquil, like sleep. Yet the racing of her heart was an autonomous response—beyond her ego's control—to Erickson's original suggestion that she be "thoroughly uncooperative." It is this aspect of her behavior—*an automatic or autono-*

mous responsiveness to suggestion which is outside the ego's control—that is actually the essence of hypnotic suggestion.

The fact that Bernice cannot even put her hand down because "it doesn't seem very natural" ratifies that she was in fact in trance—a state of autonomous responsiveness to suggestion—without any conscious understanding of her condition.

This sort of "resistance trance," wherein the patient's unconscious manifest behavior that is contrary to conscious understandings, is a fairly common form of so-called anxious resistance against hypnosis. Such patients prove themselves to be under the spell of the hypnotic situation by manifesting Baudouin's Law of Reversed Effort: the more they *try* to resist, the more they fall into a hypnotic state.[17]

"Goal-Defined" Dissociation

Automatic Writing, Anesthesia, and Amnesia

Now let's discuss this matter of dissociation. Dr. Brody has a patient who can develop a state of regression wherein she writes automatically with one hand at one age of regression and with the other hand at another age of regression. Dr. Brody, can she also talk while she is writing?

Dr. Brody: I don't know. We haven't tried it.

E: But there is that [bi-level] automatic writing—regressed at one level with one hand and regressed to another level with the other hand. There is that matter of dissociation. And, you see, the hypnotic subject can do all those things we encounter in medicine and in dentistry which the patient feels he has lost control of. In hypnosis the patient has control and is carrying out goal-directed behavior. Just think about the hysterical anesthesia. That is an anesthesia that is out of control, serving no good purpose. Hysterical amnesia is an amnesia that serves no good purpose, and it is out of control; hypnotic subjects, however, can develop those same conditions but in goal-defined situations that are under their control.

Trance Deepening and Muscular Relief

Building a Cycle of Mutually Reinforcing Contingent Suggestions

[Erickson now brings Margie, the woman he addressed in the morning session, up on stage. Bernice also remains on stage, and Erickson demonstrates multiple induction techniques.]

E: Now, Bernice, I would like to have you awaken. Wake up, wide awake. Thoroughly.

B: I just felt like I drifted off.

E: You just felt like you drifted off. That is right, and you can drift off again, can't you? Will you sit over there.

Margie, will you come up, please? Just sit down, Margie. And, Bernice, as you sit here I would like to have you go into an exceedingly deep trance; and do you mind if the audience knows what you said to me earlier today?

B: No, not a bit.

E: All right. Now listen, Bernice. As you sit here I would like to have you slowly, gradually shift and alter your muscular balance so that your back becomes increasingly comfortable and at ease; and *the more at ease you feel the deeper into the trance you go; and the deeper into trance you go, the more easily you alter the feeling in your back.* And so go very deeply into the trance, Bernice, and thoroughly enjoy the trance, because your back begins to feel better.

Trance Awakening Techniques

Suggestions for Eye Closure to "Awaken" from an Open-Eyed Trance Experience

E: Now, Margie, when did you go into a trance?

M: I don't know.

E: You don't know. I was talking to Bernice. Did you know that?

M: What? Huh? I'm sorry.

E: It's all right. You are in a trance, Margie, and so is Bernice. Bernice is going deeper and deeper. What are some of the things you would like to do, Margie?

M: I would like to learn.

E: You would like to learn. All right. I am going to ask you, Margie, to awaken. I am going to ask you to awaken shortly, and I want you to stay as wide awake as you were on the way here this morning, because I want to give you a waking task to do. Can you do that? All right, close your eyes. That is right. Breathe deeply.

If you have any question about that last part, I will explain. Very, very often your subjects don't know that they are asleep; they don't know that they are in a trance because they have their eyes open. But *they awaken much more easily and much more comfortably if you tell them to close their eyes, sleep deeply, and then awaken.*

E: Now, Margie, I want you to awaken as wide awake as you were on the way here this morning. Wake up, Margie.

M: I am with you.

Autohypnotic Induction via a Hallucinated "Joe"

E: Margie, earlier today I raised the question to the audience of how they could develop a technique for letting themselves go into autohypnotic trances. I think you were probably in a trance yourself at that point, but suppose you illustrate that technique to the audience right now. Stay awake.

M: I have to think about it to go into a trance.

E: You just have to think about it, but I described a technique of telling my friend, Joe,* sitting there in the chair, to go into a trance. A somnambulistic patient. I don't even know if you know what I mean by hand levitation. Do you?

M: Yes.

E: Suppose you talk to Joe over there.

M: Oh! I remember. Yes, you mean that little fellow who wasn't here! [Margie recalls how to give instructions to Joe to levitate "his" hand and as she does so, her voice slows and she goes into a trance.]

E: Joe went into a trance, didn't he? And Joe went into a trance, didn't he? Yes, that is right. Joe went into a trance, but you also see that Margie went into a trance, too. And you are very much amused by that, aren't you, Margie?

> Eds: This is another example of the ideodynamic principle of hypnosis: the ideas and associations aroused within Margie as she gives suggestions for the hand levitation of an imaginary subject can be sufficient to evoke a hypnotic state within her—particularly when she has an expectation

Editors' Note: This refers to a hallucinated "friend," not to the real person called Joe who previously acted as a demonstration subject.

for it which "piggybacks" off of Erickson's trance expectations for her.[18]

Facilitating a "Spontaneous" Hallucinatory Experience

Questions, Not Knowing, and Implication; Protecting and Assuring the Subject's Defenses to Deepen Trance and Catalepsy

M: I know it.

E: You know it. That is right. Do you know where you are, Margie?

M: Town and Country.

E: Listen, Margie, do you mind sitting on the beach there? Let's toss stones into the water.

M: The water.

E: Yes. Let's sit on the beach and toss stones into the water. I think that would be fun, don't you?

M: Yes.

E: Alright. You know, the sand is very nice. Is that a sailboat out there?—I mean way out there. Is that a sailboat out there?

M: I don't know.

E: You don't know. You know I am just a visitor here. I don't know the name of this beach, do you?

M: I am afraid of the water.

E: You are afraid of the water. You can't swim very well. Well, we won't go in the water, but is that a sailboat out there?

M: [I don't know.]

E: You don't know. Maybe it will come in closer and we will be able to see it; and how about tossing that stone there.

M: *How can I toss a stone when I can't move my hand!*

E: I think you can. How can you talk so silly, and you can't move your hand. I think you can.

M: *I don't understand.*

E: You are in the sand and you don't see stones. I am sorry, I thought there were stones there. But it is sand. That is right. Yes.

M: Perhaps I should go down further.

E: Perhaps you should go down further. Let us stay here for a little while. I like the look of the water down here.

M: I am afraid of it.

E: You are afraid of it. I'm not afraid. I really like it. Aren't you glad I like it?

M: Yes.

E: It is so nice to splash in the water. It is so nice for me.

M: You may have it!

E: All of it. All right, and you know that is the way I feel about fraternities and sororities. You can have them! I don't like fraternities and sororities. Anybody who wants them can have them, and that includes that attitude of pinning.

M: Yes. I don't like to pin things.

E: You don't like to pin things.

M: I don't like to pin my name on me.

E: You don't like to pin your name on you.

M: No. Do you? You will laugh.

E: Why will I laugh? Is it amusing?

M: It is a funny reason, but it is all right for me.

E: For a funny reason, it is all right for you.

M: Yes.

E: *Would it be all right for other strangers to know your reason?*

M: Yes.

E: What is the reason?

M: I feel if people want to know my name they can ask.

E: Oh! They can ask. But do you like pins?

M: No.

E: Can you tell strangers what the reason is?

M: [Response lost in the recording]

E: [Response lost in the recording]

M: It is funny.

E: You know, sometimes people drop things in the sand.

M: Yes.

E: Do you suppose there are any pins here in the sand?

M: I don't know.

E: Do you care?

M: No.

E: We'll find out if we sit on them the wrong way!

M: I will be terrified. Too early for me.

E: Why do you think I'm funny?

M: You don't miss anything.

E: I don't miss anything. What do you mean by that?

M: I just think you are humorous.

E: You think I am humorous.

M: Yes.

E: And do you know what my children say? Dad and his corn.

Eds: This is a typical example of how Erickson evokes hallucinatory experience in an appropriate subject: he simply initiates a discussion which implies that certain sensory experiences are present, and then asks questions which enable the subject to confirm the ongoing reality of the hallucination. Highly characteristic of this type of hallucinatory experience is the manifestation of the subject's own individuality—such as Margie's fear of the water. It is therefore an important part of the hypnotic art to continue to structure the hallucinatory situation in such a way as to avoid trauma while facilitating a constructive and positive experience.

It is interesting to note how Margie indicates the development of a spontaneous catalepsy when she says, "How can I toss a stone when I can't move my hand!" When Erickson tries to insist that she can move her hand, she can only reply: "I don't understand." She thereby demonstrates the state of *not knowing* which is highly typical of deep trance subjects in the process of experiencing hypnotic phenomena. Why did Margie develop this motor inhibition? Since Erickson did not explore the issue, we can only speculate. Did her fear of the hallucinated water make her grab onto whatever hypnotic defense she could produce? She had just witnessed Bernice demonstrating catalepsy. Did Margie now copy that behavior for her own defense?

Since this demonstration is taking place in front of an audience, Erickson is careful to ask, "Would it be all right for other strangers to know your reason?" Erickson was always fully respectful of the subject's individuality; the more profound or deep the trance, the more careful and protective were his actions. There is an obvious, overriding ethical reason for such care, of course. But there is also the practical professional fact that patients will only relinquish their defenses if the hypnotherapist does a good enough job of protecting them *so that they do not need to defend themselves.*

Self Hallucination

An Effort to Achieve Age Regression, Amnesia, and Dissociation; Positive Expectancy Facilitating the Summation of Minimal Therapeutic Components

E: By the way, do you know what day this is?

M: Saturday.

E: Do you mind if I change the day, the year, the month?

M: No.

E: This is 1957—March, 1957. [It is actually February, 1958.] It is Saturday, and shortly you are going to awaken on a Saturday in March, 1957. And awaken in March, 1957. Saturday. Wake up. What is the date?

M: 1957.

E: Who am I?

M: Dr. Erickson.

E: How do you know?

M: I just know.

E: You just know.

M: I have met you before.

E: Where?

M: At a dental meeting. I couldn't have met you before, could I?

E: It isn't [likely].

M: I can't think of what day it is.

E: Well, what day is it? What day is it?

M: I know it. I can't think of it.

E: What day is it?

M: Sunday.

E: No. By the way, I notice you are not wearing your name. Don't you think we should pin it on?

M: No.

E: I think so, don't you?

M: I don't know where it is.

E: We can make one.

M: Why?

E: Because everyone else is wearing one.

M: One of my usual peculiarities.

E: Well, that is easily corrected.

M: You can correct it if you like, but I thought of enjoying it.

E: *How about going swimming this evening?*

M: I will go, but *I'm afraid*.

E: You will go, but you are afraid. Don't look like that. *I want you to see somebody in the pool there. That is a nice swimming pool, isn't it?* A very nice swimming pool. They painted the walls of that swimming pool beautifully. It gives the water a new look, doesn't it? It is a large pool, isn't it? And look at that girl over there at the far side of the pool with her back toward us. *That is a striking bathing suit she has on.*

M: *I can't see—*

E: Look over there, and she is slowly turning around. Her name is Margie. That is Margie. That is Margie in the water. That is Margie.

M: In the water.

E: Yes, but look, that is Margie there. That is Margie, and she is coming here. *She is getting out of the pool very slowly. She is coming out of the pool very slowly, and pretty soon she will be way over here*, and she will climb up and be out of the water; *and she will be so glad that she is out, and she'll really be glad she is out.* That is right, and she will be so glad when she is out of that bathing suit and dressed and just sitting in the chair with her hands in her lap. *And so she will be sitting comfortably* in the chair—dressed, at ease, and then she will wake up. Wake up. Are you awake at all, Margie?

M: [Response lost in the recording.]

E: Absolutely nothing. By the way, did anybody tell you that they told me that you are afraid of pins? Are you?

M: I am not afraid of them. I just don't like them.

E: Just don't like them. They are all right in an emergency. Don't like water either.

M: Not particularly.

[Approximately four lines of conversation now lost in the recording.]

Eds: Since some of this material was lost in the recording, we do not know the extent to which the subject actually experienced age regression, amnesia, dissociation, and the self hallucination that Erickson was obviously working for. It was typical of Erickson to approach behavioral problems and phobias by having patients visually hallucinate themselves as having already solved the problem at some time in the future.[19]

Erickson's work with Margie in this section is a bit unusual in that he is attempting to have her hallucinate herself as having completed a successful swim a year ago in the past. We can study some of Erickson's approaches in this effort at facilitating the possibility of a self hallucination. He begins with an introductory question, "How about going swimming this evening?," that focuses Margie's attention on the possibility. Since she answers, "I am afraid," he cautiously encourages the possibility that she can see "somebody" in a "very nice swimming pool." Here Erickson is attempting to create as inviting and beautiful an environment as possible, and he continues with, "That is a striking bathing suit she has on." Margie replies, "I can't see—," so Erickson realizes that he must give her more time to create the hallucination. He facilitates this by carefully structuring her would-be hallucination: "Look over there, and she is *slowly* turning around ... She is getting out of the pool *very slowly*. She is coming out of the pool *very slowly,* and *pretty soon she will be way over here...* " He slows down the action and puts it into the future to give her psycho-neuro-physiological apparatus time to create the hallucinatory experience.

Notice how Erickson then utilizes her fear of water to further motivate the hallucination with "and she *will be so glad* that she is out, and *she'll really be glad* she is out ...

And so she will be sitting comfortably..." The positive feelings of being *glad* to be out of the water and *sitting comfortably* are a positive reinforcement for experiencing the visual hallucination—or at least for believing she has a memory of it from the past. The basic ideodynamic principle of hypnosis assures us that even if the subject does not fully experience the hallucination as "real," it is real at some level within the conscious-unconscious system, however minimal. (Simply describing a past life situation verbally tends to evoke some psycho-neuro-physiological experience of it.) Because of this basic ideodynamic principle, Erickson was not discouraged when a subject failed to fall completely under the spell of an hallucinatory experience. Erickson always assumed that some components of the experience were activated, even if the subject's conscious mind denied it. Often these minimal components of the experience remained active within a patient's unconscious, slowly building a therapeutic potential without the patient's conscious awareness of it. When Erickson had activated enough of these minimal components, they would "summate" and present the patient's conscious mind with a dramatic and apparently sudden therapeutic change. *Erickson's positive attitude of expectancy for a therapeutic outcome* was often the only source of reinforcement for the "minimal therapeutic components," which usually summated within the patient's unconscious without any help from the discouraged conscious mind.

Turning Failure into Success

The Sudden Summation of Minimal Unconscious Therapeutic Components as the Basis of "Faith Healing" and "Miraculous Cures"

E: Do you know, Margie, when you want somebody to do something in using hypnosis—especially if you are a medical man, a dentist, or an experimenter in a psychology labora-

tory—it is quite important to try to get the person to do a task, and so you set it up for them to fail.

M: Why?

E: Why? Because *anybody who fails also wants to succeed. You set up one task and you bring about a failure; at the same time, you are also motivating a very great desire for success.*

That is one of the techniques that I want to impress upon you. Now certainly all of you recognize that Margie has a profound amnesia for pins and for water, and for all the attendant circumstances of the entire situation. Yes, she doesn't like water, and, yes, she doesn't like pins; and so I dealt with something that is definitely painful to her in some way.

> Eds: Because our transcript is incomplete, we cannot find the evidence for Erickson's statement, "Margie has a profound amnesia for pins and for water." However we can observe one of his interesting maneuvers and insights into failure and success when he says, "You set up one task and you bring about failure; at the same time you are also motivating a very great desire for success." Is Erickson simply being something of a scoundrel here by attempting to turn the apparent failure of his demonstration into a success by rationalizing that failure actually motivates success? Or does every failure indeed evoke fresh, minimal unconscious components for eventual success?! Might the sudden summation of these motivational and therapeutic components also serve as the basis of the seemingly miraculous cures brought about by faith healers, psychics, shaman, etc? By projecting the power of success onto another, the patient depotentiates his own barriers of belief in failure and unknowingly gives "free reign" to those intrinsic elements of healing which are needed for the "cure." The cure then appears to be mediated by another person, when in fact the other person only served to "carry" the

projection of success needed to activate and summate the patient's "minimal unconscious components." We see less dramatic manifestations of the same process in the phenomenon of iatrogenic disease and healing, in which the physician's negative or positive expectancy apparently alters the course of the patient's physical outcome.

Although Erickson never formally stated it as such, a strong case could be made for the view that Erickson himself regarded the careful utilization and summation of "minimal cues" as the essence of indirect suggestion and hypnotic induction. Indeed he would probably agree that they served as the actual "psycho-neuro-physiological" (Erickson's phrase) basis for hypnotherapeutic success, as well as for "miraculous cures," "mind reading," and many so-called psychic phenomenon.[20]

Associative Gaps and Distraction

Building up and Breaking Down Amnesia and Anesthesia

E: Do you wish you knew what I was talking about, Margie?

M: Yes.

E: You don't know what I am talking about. How do you think I felt when my daughter got pinned with a fraternity pin?

M: I don't know.

E: You don't know.

M: I don't know how you felt.

E: How do you think I feel about fraternities or sororities?

M: You said something about them.

E: I said something about them, didn't I?

M: You said, "They can have them; I don't like them."

E: What did I say about fraternities?

M: That they could have them.

E: Did I say that? Who could have what? Who could have what? Well, what are we talking about? The sand on the beach? My daughter?

M: How would you feel if your daughter were pinned.

E: I told her she practically began life that way.

M: I hope she has made some progress! I don't mean to be impertinent—I really don't.

We are talking about fraternities and sororities, and how to get over here. The matter of the distraction is the idea. First I can start breaking down the amnesia. Then I can distract the subject's attention and re-establish that amnesia. You must have a willingness to learn how to manipulate behavior so that you can produce an amnesia in whatever part of the memory that you want to, break it down, and then re-establish it.

The same is true in the matter of anesthesia: you can allow it to break down and build up and break down. One of the things that is so awfully important in the medical use of hypnosis is the willingness on the part of the anesthetist to reinduce a trance and re-establish anesthesia. Often a patient undergoing an operation will suddenly come out of the trance and say, "What is going on here? Ouch, that hurts!" You ought to realize that by some simple little remark, you can distract the patient's attention and successfully reinduce trance.

Overcoming a Pin Phobia

Utilizing Minimal Approaches, Implication, and Confusion

E: Do you object to holding the pin?

M: No. Just so I don't have to wear it.

E: Just so you don't have to wear it.

M: [Response lost in the recording.]

E: It wasn't really important, was it, that I put it there?

M: You just don't understand. I don't like pins. I don't like to pin something on me.

E: You don't like to pin something on you.

M: I don't like to pin my name on myself.

Now, what is the importance of that? Always in approaching a patient you make the minimal approaches.

E: You don't like your name pinned on you. You just don't.

M: I love that quirk in you.

E: That would be all right. It isn't your name. As long as it isn't your name, it is all right if I pin this. Would it be all right if I didn't pin this?

M: Yes.

E: That would be all right. Of course it is all right, but there is the pin, there is the name, and that is all right too.

M: Will it be all right if I don't?

E: That is right. I could pin this on me.

M: Yes.

E: That wouldn't be right, would it? What are you thinking?

M: What do I have in mind?

E: What do I have in mind.

Now I can't say that I could have had a nicer demonstration. It wouldn't be right to pin this card with her name on me. That is right, it wouldn't be right to pin it on me. The implication is that it should be pinned on her. That would be right, and I paused long enough so that she could begin to get a little bit of distress. But in the hypnotic situation you do not allow that time.

E: You wouldn't want me to pin this on you?

M: I don't want to try.

Just think how she followed the implication: "I don't want to try." You see her responses. Have I asked her yet? I haven't even asked her, and she is making that response.

M: I haven't.

E: You haven't. What next?

M: It's hopeless.

E: What is hopeless?

M: I suppose you want this pinned on me.

All right, and I want you to notice how she made that statement: If I want the pin on her, it's pretty hopeless; but the implication of her remark is that *I can pin it on her.*

It is no longer a question of "I don't want it"; it has slowly become a question of "If you want it, I can do it." It then becomes an action done for me, not for her. This dilutes and lessens the traumatic significance of it—whatever it is—and the patient gets the opportunity of discovering that the thing isn't so bad.

Re-Induction of Trance

Facilitating Visual Hallucination via Questions Evoking Previous Associational Networks: "Is That a Sailboat?"

E: By the way, is that a sailboat? Just answer.

M: I don't think so.

E: What do you mean, "I don't think so"?

M: I don't know what it looks like.

E: Where?

M: On the ocean.

E: What ocean?

M: The one we were in.

E: [Response lost in the recording.]

M: On the sand at the ocean.

E: We were on the sand at the ocean.

M: We weren't really on it at the ocean, but I thought we were.

E: You thought we were. Where did I get the idea we could throw stones in the water?

M: I don't know. We were in the sand.

E: We were in the sand, that is right. But we still are, aren't we? I think this is very pretty sand, don't you? Look at those gulls out there. Haven't they got a graceful flight?

M: I don't know what you are talking about.

E: The sand, the ocean, and the gulls.

M: I don't see any gulls.

E: But look. Just this side of the sailboat.

M: I don't see any gulls.

E: This side of the sailboat.

M: There isn't any sailboat.

E: Where are we?

M: I am here.

E: Look out there at the sailboat.

M: But I don't see any, I told you.

E: All right, now look at the ocean and the sailboat. That is right, and you see it out there, or isn't that a sailboat? Don't you think the gulls are graceful in their flight?

M: I don't know.

E: You don't know. You can't see the clouds, you don't know if that is a sailboat. I wish we had some stones here to put in the water, don't you?

M: I am afraid of it.

E: You are afraid of the water.

M: I'd rather stay here on the beach.

E: Here on the beach. All right. Let's not go in the water.

Now, what I wanted you to appreciate is this: a patient can show a lot of resistance and can argue, "I don't see a sailboat; I know that we are here"; but with your willingness to persist, and with your willingness to re-establish some of the associations, some of the conditionings of a previous trance, you can re-establish that trance state.

Physical Contact in Trance

The Importance of Tactile Persistence as a Conditioning Factor; Tactile Suggestions for Inducing Hand Levitation and Catalepsy

Now as I mentioned before, you may have a patient come out of anesthesia in the middle of an operation in a state of fright. I prefer to have the patient laughing at me and amused at my expense—just resisting me in that way—rather than the unpleasant frame of mind of being frightened and terrified. This is a teaching situation, but in the operating room you can handle fright and terror in exactly the same way that you handle this laughter. It is your persistence and your willingness to take hold and re-establish the trance state by a conditioned response.

Always in your work with patients, you ought to have physical contact as one aspect of the conditioning process. In the matter of touching the patient, I want all of you to bear in mind that you move a hand, you lift a hand, by the slightest kind of a touch: you suggest the movement instead of grabbing hold and hauling it around; you merely raise the hand by touching the thumb gently, smoothly, and then you move it up or you move it down by the fashion in which you stimulate the tip of the thumb with the tip of your finger. You do not suggest a catalepsy by lifting the hand and suggesting the patient maintain that position. A catalepsy achieved in that manner is too often a matter of complaisance. The way you suggest catalepsy is to take hold of the hand and then slowly minimize your touch. You can minimize the touch of your thumb on the back of the patient's hand, or you can draw your fingers out to the fingertips so that you decrease the support of your hand bit by bit, and in a graduated fashion. Then you simply leave the hand in that cataleptic position.[21]

Ratifying Trance

Dissociation and Catalepsy as Trance Indicators; Questions to Evoke Hypnotic Catalepsy; Posthypnotic Suggestion

E: Where are you, Margie?

M: At Town and Country.

E: Will you close your eyes, sleep deeply, and then awaken. Wake up. Wake up. Hi!

M: Hi.

E: Are you awake, Margie?

M: Yes.

E: You are sure of that?

M: You forgot something—to awaken my arms.

E: And that is your statement: that I forgot something. And you are so right.

But what I want the audience to appreciate is this: that there is this element known as dissociation that accounts for a great deal of hypnotic behavior, and Margie's arms are very much dissociated, and her arms can remain in a trance. That is, her unconscious can maintain a rather rigid control over her hands.

E: And, Bernice, I would like to have you take a look at that arm, and I would like to have you understand that that is the sort of thing you can apply to your back.

B: My back feels fine.

E: Your back feels fine. By the way, have you been in a trance today?

B: I don't know for sure—I hope I was, twice.

E: You don't know for sure; you hope you were twice. What are you thinking, Margie?

M: I like it.

E: You like it. *Is all the rest of you awake? Are you sure of that? I wonder, can you walk?*

M: I don't know, shall I?

E: I was just wondering. Can you walk?

M: I don't know if I want to.

E: Do you want to? How do you feel about getting up?

M: I don't know.

E: Will you personally ask her to stand up, Dr. Brodie?

Dr. B: Margie, would you please stand up—for me? *Try and stand up for me.*

M: I can't, I really can't.

E: Well, tell him why.

M: I don't know.

E: *Try real hard.*

M: I'm too heavy.

E: You are too heavy.

M: I don't know why.

How many of you recognize why she can't stand up? She knows about the catalepsy of her arm, but she doesn't know about the catalepsy of her legs. And you know the first thing in getting up is the drawing back of the feet. But Margie's legs are cataleptic, although she didn't realize it. Her legs are very definitely cataleptic. You see, you always have the opportunity of testing and analyzing your patient's behavior so that you can note the interrelationships.

E: Margie, will you close your eyes and go way, deep sound asleep. And, Paul, will you close your eyes and go really sound asleep. That is right. Now I want you to rest soundly, deeply, peacefully. I want it to feel like eight hours of solid rest, and then I want you to awaken feeling rested and refreshed and energetic. And, Joe, I want you to know that any time you want to go into a deep trance, you can and you will—any time you want to. And, Bernice, I want you to realize that you can go into a deep trance any time you wish. All right, wake up, Margie. Wake up, Paul. Wake up, Joe. Bernice, are you awake?

B: I am trying.

> Eds: In this interesting section Margie first informs Erickson that he has forgotten to awaken her arms. This was her way of describing the experience of catalepsy or dissociation whereby she cannot move a part of her body. Surely this is an indication that she is still in an altered state, even though she has just verbally indicated that she is awake. Erickson takes this occasion to give an intellectual aside to the audience about the phenomenon of dissociation. His comments also function as an indirect suggestion to Bernice that her unconscious can do the same thing to help her with her back problem. He then turns to Bernice to give her the same suggestion in a direct manner, and she responds that her back "feels fine."
>
> Next Erickson presents a series of questions to Margie: "Is all the rest of you awake? Are you sure of that? I wonder, can you walk?" All these questions are designed to make Margie wonder and then doubt whether she is fully awake, and whether she can walk. The hypnotic suggestion implied in these questions is that *she is not awake* and that *she cannot walk*. In fact, *she cannot even stand up.* She does not even know why she is "too heavy." *Feeling heavy,* of course, is actually just another way some people experience the deep relaxation that is characteristic of this form of trance.
>
> Erickson then concludes the demonstration with all the subjects in his typical fashion: by giving suggestions for eye closure, deep sleep, and a refreshed and energetic awakening. Bernice, however, is still having trouble awakening—another trance indicator—even though she is "trying."

115

QUESTIONS AND ANSWERS

Thumbsucking

Prescribing the Symptom: Paradoxical or Reverse Suggestion and Reframing

Q. Can you suggest a simple, short treatment procedure for mild thumbsucking in young children?

A. You develop that willingness to praise the child for sucking his thumb. One of the first lessons the child gets in life is: you must take your turn on this and that. And, you know, the right thumb needs a turn at sucking just as the left thumb needs a turn at sucking; and the little finger needs a turn, and the other little finger, and the forefinger, and the middle finger. And you give each finger a turn, and you do a nice job; and you praise the child for it, and soon it all gets so tiresome.

I know one little boy who told his grandmother, "This is making me dislike sucking my thumb!" And she asked him what he would like to do when he cooled off. He said, "A lot of other things!" That is right, but he himself gave his own prognosis. It is that simple technique of encouraging the child in his own bad habit.

Q. How often do you usually need to see a child [you are treating with this type of procedure]?

A. You educate the parents. I see the child two, three, maybe four times, and praise him properly. See to it that the parents cooperate. See to it that the child takes turns [sucking each and every finger].

> Eds: Erickson's *utilization approaches* to thumbsucking are described in more detail in Volume I of *Collected Papers*, and in *Healing in Hypnosis*, (Volume I of this series). The point is that the child soon gets tired of having to suck all ten fingers, and so gives up sucking the thumb as well.

As is the case with most of Erickson's interventions in habit problems, this case could be conceptualized as prescribing the symptom, paradoxical suggestion or reframing. It is a paradoxical or reverse suggestion "to praise the child for sucking his thumb," and it is a process of reframing to view the situation as one of "giving equal attention to all fingers" rather than "giving up thumbsucking." In either case the therapeutic outcome was a dissipation of the habit out of sheer inconvenience.

Medication and Placebos in Hypnosis

Q. What do you think about the use of medication as an aid in using hypnosis with more difficult subjects?

A. Personally, I don't like the use of medication. I have tried everything. The only drug I think is at all good is about an ounce of C_2H_5OH [ethyl alcohol—whiskey] about half an hour in advance. Sometimes by the operator, sometimes by the patient! All kidding aside, I don't think much of drugs as an aid. If the patient insists on drugs the best to use is a placebo. If you use a drug, you are then dealing with a patient plus drug effects. Therefore, use a placebo whenever possible.

Superior Judgment of the Unconscious

Q. What about getting the unconscious to do work? Does this use of energy on an unconscious level interfere with the total energy available? In other words, could working with the unconscious in hypnosis injure the patient if done too frequently?

A. As soon as you start abusing yourself, the unconscious is very likely to make you overpoweringly sleepy and you will then go to sleep on the job. But you aren't likely to strain yourself nearly as much as when you use your own conscious, often poor, judgment. Your unconscious mind uses much better judgment than your conscious mind.

Treating Insomnia via Arithmetical Progression

Q. Would you describe a short technique for treating a patient with insomnia? How often should the patient be seen?

A. I'll give an example of one of the techniques I like to use in treating insomnia. A man came to me and said: "I sleep only two hours a night. I go to sleep when that clock in my bedroom strikes one, and I wake up when it strikes three."

Nothing on earth could induce him to take that clock out of his bedroom. I took practically an hour to laboriously explain to him this matter of arithmetical progression, and he finally agreed to sleep 2 hours and 1 minute, then 2 hours-1 minute-1 second, 2 hours-1 minute-2 seconds, then -4 seconds, -8, -16, -32, -64 seconds, and up to 2 hours and 2 minutes. And when we had built it up in this fashion he said, "Why not build it up by minutes instead of by seconds?" So we finally agreed that he could sleep any reasonable number of hours—anywhere from 6 hours a night to 10 hours a night, probably averaging between 7 1/2 to 8 hours of sleep.

Now my technique was first to get him to accept that concept of arithmetical progression, and then to acknowledge that it really didn't make any difference whether he slept 2 hours, or 2 hours and 1 second. Getting him to accept that one second constituted a therapeutic victory. So often that is your case, whether you are giving an anesthesia for the correction of insomnia or for the correction of neurosis.

Treating Headaches

Degree of Symptom Removal Determined by Degree of Patient's Motivation

Q. How helpful is self-hypnosis for a person who is inclined to develop melancholia following a nervous breakdown? And can hypnosis be useful in controlling headaches where there is apparently no physiological reason for them?

A. I would suggest psychiatric aid for melancholia following a nervous breakdown.

In the matter of autohypnosis for a headache of psychological origin, you have to consider the willingness on the part of the patient to have the headache. You had better recognize that a lot of symptomatology is demanded by the total personality via a willingness to have the symptom. [Once you recognize this point,] your question to the patient becomes: "How long do you want to have that headache? Are you willing to have a headache for 2 or 3 seconds?; willing to have a headache for 2 or 3 minutes?"

I had one patient who was bedridden about three months out of the year by severe headaches. She lost all that time; was never able to agree to any social function because she didn't know when she would have a headache. She was only willing to see me four times, and all I could do for her was to settle it in this way: she now has a headache every Monday morning, which is usually the most convenient time. It is a rather severe headache lasting all of 60 whole seconds, even up to 90 whole seconds. It is very severe pain. She lies down in bed, has her headache, then gets up. Sometimes she even has to postpone the headache until Tuesday.

There is that willingness to have the headache, and the patient may not be willing to lose it through all the psychotherapy that may be required. But the patient's willingness to have the headache implies a willingness to control it. The patient who comes to you and says, "I don't want even the slightest vestige of any of my symptomatology," is a patient who is offering you a rather difficult problem.

Catharsis in Trance and Waking States

Treating the Conscious and Unconscious as Separate "Individuals"

Q. Once you have performed some sort of catharsis for a patient in a trance state, is it good to go over the situation in an awakened state in order to fortify the results?

A. I think it is awfully important for a patient who has undergone a trance experience of a therapeutic sort—undergone a catharsis—to understand that experience in the trance state; and then in the trance state you also ought to tell him that he is going to need to remember the experience in the waking state, and that he ought to choose the time and the situation. You can point out the desirability of your office, or the next appointment—whatever it is—but you help him understand that he must also repeat the catharsis in the waking state. You can comfort him by pointing out that he can do as Margie did: have that arm dissociated so that all the rest of her was awake, but not her arm. So it is with the waking catharsis: experience that part of the trauma that can be tolerated by the conscious mind, and then later experience an additional part, and still later yet another part, until the trauma has been completed. Then you put the patient back in the trance state and acquaint him with the fact that he has had a catharsis, both in the trance state and in the waking state. Finally you awaken him and let him be aware of the fact that he has had the catharsis both in the waking state and in the trance state. In other words, *you treat the unconscious mind and the conscious mind as two separate individuals that are functioning for the good of one person.*

Psychological Control of Physiological Functions

Utilizing Experiential Learnings from Everyday Life

Q. What is your theory or explanation of the hypnotic control of what we consider normal physiological functioning such as bleeding or salivation?

A. Suppose you are a college student. Today is your birthday, and you are looking out your window and down the street to see if the postman is coming. You've been promised a book, but you also start licking your chops and drooling because you know there is a good chance he also may bring some candy. Now a long time ago you learned to associate candy with salivation, and so you drool at the sight of the postman who is your only contact with home. You are drooling at the sight of the postman because he reminds you of your birthday possibilities, and you have a life-long experience of responding at a physiological level to a lot of psychological forces.

Now most of you are not aware of [this interrelationship of physiological and psychological forces]. In your present type of thinking, you do not believe, for example, that you could control the flow of blood; that you could cut down on bleeding. Yet you all know that the utterance of one single word right now could bring a flush to the face of all of you. And that is right, because your body has had a lot of experience in controlling the flow of blood, and it is so easy and so simple. And if you can control the flow of blood in your face, well, why shouldn't you be able to control it in your neck; and your neck does turn red and your forehead does turn red, and why not a little bit below. And consider the way in which your body has had experience in turning pale at the thought of something terrifying, and consider the way your body has had many experiences in turning red under heat and turning white under cold. Your body has had a lot of experience; there is a tremendous wealth of actual physiological experience that warrants the expectation that one could build up a hypnotic situation to control capillary flow of blood; and with that capillary flow of blood you could also control salivary glands, or you could stimulate those glands. You can say a single word to someone that will produce tears. Those tears require an alteration of the flow of blood in the tear glands, and you don't even know how those tear glands are supplied with blood. There is a *wealth of knowledge that exists in your body,* of which you are totally unaware, and that will manifest itself when given the right psychological or physiological stimulation.

> Eds: This "wealth of knowledge that exists in your body" is formed by all the automatic and unconscious conditioned responses that occur when psychological and physiological states are associated in the normal course of living. Erickson usually referred to this phenomenon as "experiential learning" and considered it the raw material out of which hypnotic responses could be elicited.[22]

Producing Localized Anesthesia for Dental Purposes

Q. How can a rapid anesthesia of one tooth be accomplished?

A. I wouldn't attempt the rapid anesthesia of just one tooth. But I would be perfectly willing to tell the patient that, and then settle for a rapid anesthesia of all the teeth in that side of his mouth. Next I would teach him that this is the tooth I want, and I would use a thoroughly good distraction technique which I usually devise in accordance with the immediate situation. If I were to work with a particular patient—on Gale, for example—I would certainly try to distract his attention by pointing out to him that perhaps I could pinch him on the shoulder. That isn't what he wants; he wants an absence of pain in the left side of his mandible. I would ask him to agree to [be pinched on the shoulder, and in that way] start to produce the generalized anesthesia.

Hypnosis and Learning

Improving Study Incentives; Ethical Considerations in Preserving the Patient's Personal Rights

Q. Can incentive be improved in a junior high school boy who simply will not study?

A. Whenever you try to use hypnosis for a purely selfish purpose, you lose. I can think of the doctor who was very pleased with his son, Johnny, who was a prized hypnotic subject. Johnny was twelve years old. Then Johnny brought his report card home, and there was one D, plenty of C's, and one B. Papa put Johnny in a trance and explained to him that he had to get some B's and A's. Then Papa discovered that Johnny wouldn't go into a trance for him ever again, because, you see, Papa tried to use hypnosis to make Johnny do Papa's bidding. That is wrong; it is unfair; it is unjust. It is a violation of Johnny; it is a violation of Johnny's unconscious.

I pointed out to the father that I could raise Johnny's grades, but that I would do it in a different way. I put Johnny in a trance and said: "Johnny, your father tried to tell you that you had to have all A's and B's. Let us be honest about this; let us be fair and decent. Johnny, you didn't feel too badly about the D, did you? You didn't think it was important. You didn't feel too badly about the C's; they are perfectly good grades; they are average grades. And you really did enjoy the B grade, didn't you?"

And Johnny did enjoy his B grade. Now that is where I stopped. I approved of his good grade. I approved of his C grade, and I pointed out sympathetically that he didn't mind the D grade too much, and that is what he thought I believed. So he raised his grades because he didn't want any more sympathy about his D's, be he *did* want the emotional satisfaction of more B's—but that was *his* want. I just told him it was all right to enjoy B's, so he started out getting more B's. To tell him, as his father had, "You ought to get more A's," would have been an unjustifiable intrusion upon Johnny's personal rights.

The Case of Robert's Traumatic Truck Accident

Treating Nightmares in Children by Active Participation, Elaboration and Reframing

Q. Do you have a solution for alarming nightmares?

A. My son Robert was hit by a truck when he was seven years old. Both thighs were broken, his pelvis was fractured, he had a brain concussion, and a few other sordid bits of damage. When he got home from the hospital with his body cast on, he began to have nightmares—horrible nightmares. I sat on his bed and listened to his screaming; I listened to the words he used through one nightmare after another until I knew the words thoroughly, and I knew the order in which he would scream. In this way I learned the content and sequence of that nightmare: there is a truck coming; it is going to hit me; it is going to kill me; oh! and then his collapse.

I did the following once I knew the sequence, the next time

Robert had his nightmare. As soon as he started screaming, "There is a truck coming!," I agreed, "There is a truck coming, and it is getting closer and closer." Then I just speeded up his nightmare [so that he came more quickly to the point of] "Oh!," and his collapse. Soon Robert became a bit dependent on my joining in that nightmare, and then it became possible for me to say, "There is another truck coming, but it is on the other side of the street." So I introduced another element into his nightmare, namely, another truck on the other side of the street. Still later I was able to introduce the idea that the truck on the other side of the street would miss him. As soon as I had that idea adequately implanted, I said, "The truck is going to hit you, but you are going to get well." At that point I had the nightmare pretty well whipped. After a few more weeks of this procedure Robert had his nightmare with all of my emendations and corrections and additions, and with the realization that he didn't have to have any more nightmares.

And with other children I have always corrected their nightmares by telling them: "Yes, you did have this, you did have that," and I join in. For you'd better join in, and you'd better use undesirable elements in order to get control of the nightmare. Any effort to have reassured Robert would have been contrary to fact. The truck had hit him, and therefore I abided by that fact. The idea is to join in and elaborate and extend and improve understanding.

Contraindications in Dental Hypnosis

Recognizing Disruptive Personality Disturbances

Q. Would you suggest contraindications for the use of hypnosis in dentistry? Are there any signs of unfavorable conditions that the dentist should recognize in the patient?

A. When I consider how difficult it is for me to recognize a potential psychotic patient when he first comes into my office, I am at a loss to suggest to dentists—who do not have psychiatric training—those personality disturbances that contraindicate hypnosis. I am very much at a loss, because it is only in the very obvious cases that immediate recognition is possible. I have seen some awfully nice, sweet people in my office. I studied them, I thought them over, and I missed the goal entirely—because all of a sudden they developed an acute psychosis. And yet when I first saw these patients there was no real evidence of psychosis that I could detect. So my general tendency, no matter who enters my office, is to look at the person and wonder just how soon he or she will be committed—until I can answer that question for myself as accurately as possible. In general, when [extreme conditions are] perfectly obvious, avoid hypnosis; but otherwise, you are going to miss the mark just as many times as I do.

Treating Sexual Problems

Psychological Reorientation and Reframing

Q. Would you approach the treatment of frigidity or impotence with direct suggestions if the patient refused psychological orientation?

A. I wouldn't try any direct suggestion. In fact, I wouldn't use hypnosis to correct the impotence or the frigidity, because both impotence and frigidity are rather deeply involved problems employing faulty attitudes toward the body, faulty orientations toward the body, and a lot of confused understanding on the subject of sex and emotion in general. Therefore, I would use the hypnosis for the purpose of providing a different psychological orientation.[23]

The Role of Confidence in Successful Trance Induction

Q. How important is the competence of the hypnotist in producing a trance in subjects?

A. In the vast majority of cases, it is the competence you are willing to radiate that enables you to induce hypnosis. It is your willingness to know that you can do it. I carried on experiments with medical students wherein I told one group of students that this particular subject was a very poor subject and had failed miserably, while I told another group of students that the same individual was an excellent subject and that they would succeed in the induction.

After the experiment, about every other one of these medical students said, "I tried as hard as I could but I couldn't induce a trance in that subject." What was really the problem? They lacked confidence. My assertion to this group had been that the subject was just no good, just impossible, and because of that awareness or belief they lacked confidence. But the students whom I had told, "The subject is an excellent one; goes into a trance easily; develops anesthesia easily," had utter confidence and they got the good results. Now, if you can achieve such results experimentally, you can also achieve such results in your own practices. I think you ought to have confidence and trust in your own professional capacities.

Remembering Versus Forgetting

Determining the Desirability of Amnesia Versus Memory for Trance Events

Q. When is it best to suggest to the patient either amnesia or complete memory for the trance?

A. I always tell patients, "You can remember this or you can forget this as you wish"; or, [if I don't tell them that directly,] I somehow imply it. My statement usually centers around the idea that "Whatever it is you need to understand consciously or unconsciously, that is what I want you to understand. In other words, I want you to understand consciously whatever you need to; I want you to understand unconsciously whatever you need to." Thus I place the onus of responsibility on the patients' shoulders. If they need to understand 75 percent of the trance experience on an unconscious level, then they get a 75 percent amnesia.

Hypnosis in the Treatment of Compulsions

Q. Can hypnosis be used for the compulsive drinker or smoker?

A. Hypnosis is often used with the compulsive patient, and it is probably best employed by utilizing the compulsion. With the compulsive smoker, for example, you can build up quite easily, quite gently, a compulsion to quit smoking, a compulsion to lose the taste for smoking.

I can think of a doctor in Chicago who was a compulsive smoker. He smoked four to six packs of cigarettes a day, and he really suffered if he didn't have that second cigarette ready to stick in his mouth as soon as he discarded the finished one. My statement to him was, "You really need to have full packs of cigarettes in your pockets, don't you?" I built up that compulsion, and then I built up the second compulsion: "You don't know on what day you are going to quit smoking. You don't know whether it will be the first part of July, the middle part of July, or the last part of July; but you are pretty darned sure it will happen before the 15th of August, and you would give your soul to know the day."

So my patient developed a tremendous compulsion to know on what day he was going to quit smoking, but it *had* to be before the 15th of August because he just couldn't wait that long to know!

In September he said to me: "That was a smart trick you played on me. You made me so compulsively interested in quitting smoking that I just couldn't wait for the day; so I jumped the gun. I could have held out until the middle of August, but I didn't; I quit around the 20th of July, and now this is September."

I saw him again in October and he still hadn't smoked. "You know," he said, "I still have a compulsion about cigarettes." He reached into his pocket and hauled out a pack. "I have a compulsion to carry around a full pack of cigarettes. I don't dare open it because then it might not be a full pack. I don't mind that extra load."

So he carries a full pack. A compulsive need. I asked him how he felt about that use of his compulsion. He said: "It is fine with me. Four to six packs of cigarettes a day meant I ought to get my head examined. This way I can get my pocket examined!"

Neurodermatitis

Hypnotic Treatment via Psychological Reorientation: Partial Symptom Removal: "How Much Do You Need to Keep?"

Q. Is hypnosis useful in the treatment of neurodermatitis?

A. In the treatment of neurodermatitis you have the psychological reaction to the actual organic problem, and you have the personality reaction to it; so you use hypnosis to redefine the amount of neurodermatitis that the patient actually needs on a purely organic basis. I had one patient who had been tutored through grade school and high school because he was in bed, literally, all that time. Now and then he would have a month or six weeks of remission. He came to me during one such remission period, and my entire therapy for his neurodermatitis centered around this idea:

"Just how much of this neurodermatitis do you need to keep? Obviously the Mayo Clinic can't be wrong; all the other clinics you went to can't be wrong. But you do react psychologically and as a personality. Now, how much of this neurodermatitis do you need to keep, because there is no cure for it?" The patient settled for a patch on the forehead, on the neck, on the wrist, on the elbow, and on the anterior surface of both thighs. And when he gets mad at this or that he gets a patch on his chest; but when he *really really really* gets mad he develops a hand-sized patch on his abdomen. He had had a terrific patch on his abdomen when his girl jilted him, so he saves his abdomen for the really really really mad times. In just ordinary mad times, his chest is enough. He has very little neurodermatitis now. He graduated *summa cum laude* from college; he was a fraternity president and an outstanding student—the first time in his life he ever really went to school!

Pruritis

Hypnotic Treatment via Reframing: the "Calloused Nerves" Pseudo-Concept

Q. In handling a case of pain and/or pruritis, do you try to displace the sensation with another symptom, decrease the intensity in the affected areas, or what?

A. Let us take the condition of pruritis since the treatment of pain follows the same general pattern. You ask the patient to be forthright and direct and straightforward about admitting his pruritis. You ask him to discuss it in utter detail and with absolute frankness so that he can recognize that it is a disability just as an aching tooth is a disability, or an abscess, an earache, a sore throat, or whatever.

Once you have established the pruritis on a sound medical level, then you can raise the question that perhaps last week sometime—perhaps for as long as three seconds—the pruritis let up, and so you bring up the matter of nerve fatigue. Then you can point out that perhaps the pruritis let up for a whole minute at another time. In fact, you can prove to your patient by the very intensity with which you speak to him and control his attention that it has let up while you have been talking, and only now has it returned. Just as an awareness of the shoes on his feet can come and go, you have made your dent in the patient so that he can accept the idea that the pruritis can wax and wane; it can get worse and it can get better. Now you emphasize the getting better phase and you shorten the periods of getting worse. You build up in him the concept of learning how to develop callouses on the nerves and on the end organs of nerves so that the nerves become so accustomed to the distressing pruritis that [the patient as a total personality] doesn't even notice it. You can also point out the example of the boiler-factory worker who gets so used to the noise in the factory that he talks in an ordinary conversational tone of voice to his co-workers, who reply in a similarly normal tone of voice; and they hear each other despite that infernal din.

Hypnotic Induction of Audience

Suggestions for Unconscious Review and Utilization of Lecture Learnings: Posthypnotic Suggestions for Future Autohypnotic Experiences

Q. A large number of the people here today have asked if you would do a mass induction of this group and give suggestions for the retention of all this information that you have given us today, as well as suggestions for autohypnosis?

A. I would like to suggest that you lean back in your chairs, close your eyes, and listen to me. Some of you may not be interested in going into a trance and you may know that; some of you may be interested in going into a trance but may not even dream that you are interested. Therefore all of you ought to lean back, and all of you ought to close your eyes and listen, because you can listen and stay awake if you need to with your eyes closed; but if you really want to go into a trance you can do so.

What is the technique that I need to employ for this group? I have lectured to you all day long. I have talked on the subject of hypnosis; you are very familiar with this and that technique of hypnosis. In the matter of going into a hypnotic trance, it is a matter of listening and letting something happen to you, of becoming interested in your own feeling, of recognizing that externalities are not important. As you sit there relaxed with your eyes closed, I would like to have you review some of the thoughts you had this morning. I want you to do that reviewing in your own unconscious mind; in that part of your mind that

does its thinking and its remembering and its understanding without letting you know consciously that it is doing so. I want your unconscious mind to review everything I said on the subject of fear and anxiety and the alleviation of various symptoms. I want your unconscious mind to go over all that I said. I want your unconscious mind to go over your own personal understandings of those matters, and then I want your own unconscious mind to move on to the next topics that were discussed—the questions of technique, applications of hypnosis, and all the thinking that you did.

I want you to bear in mind that some of the time you listened to me and were forgetful of your surroundings; that you were interested in your own learnings as a personality, interested in your own unconscious responses to this particular type of gathering. And I would like to have you review what took place this afternoon, particularly in regard to the trance demonstrations and your awareness that the subjects went into trances, that they achieved their own learnings, and that you achieved learnings along with them.

I want you to bear in mind that it isn't necessary for you to strive pointedly and directly to learn things. Your willingness to learn things incidentally, as part of another situation, is sufficient; there is your willingness to learn something about going into a trance for yourself by watching your own patient, by listening to your own patient, by seeing the kind of learning that your patient is achieving. I would like to have you realize that in your sleep at night, in your dreams, that you can make use of your own unconscious mind to review all of the learnings that you have acquired from your own experience, from your own practice, and all the learnings that you have acquired at various meetings and lectures.

I want you to realize that with the educational background and training that you have, all you need do is to just sit quietly in a chair, relaxing and relying upon your own unconscious mind to direct and to guide you; and it will teach you a great deal about going into an autohypnotic trance. I want you to realize that you know enough to be able to do it. So for a few minutes rest deeply and comfortably. Be interested in your own experiences as something that belongs to you, belongs to your own unconscious, to be made available to you by your unconscious whenever you need them—not necessarily by name, but by a feeling of confidence that you can do this or do that; that you can understand things as they develop. And now in just a few moments, slowly rouse up feeling rested and refreshed.

MILTON H. ERICKSON
A PHOTOGRAPHIC PORTFOLIO: 1910–1980

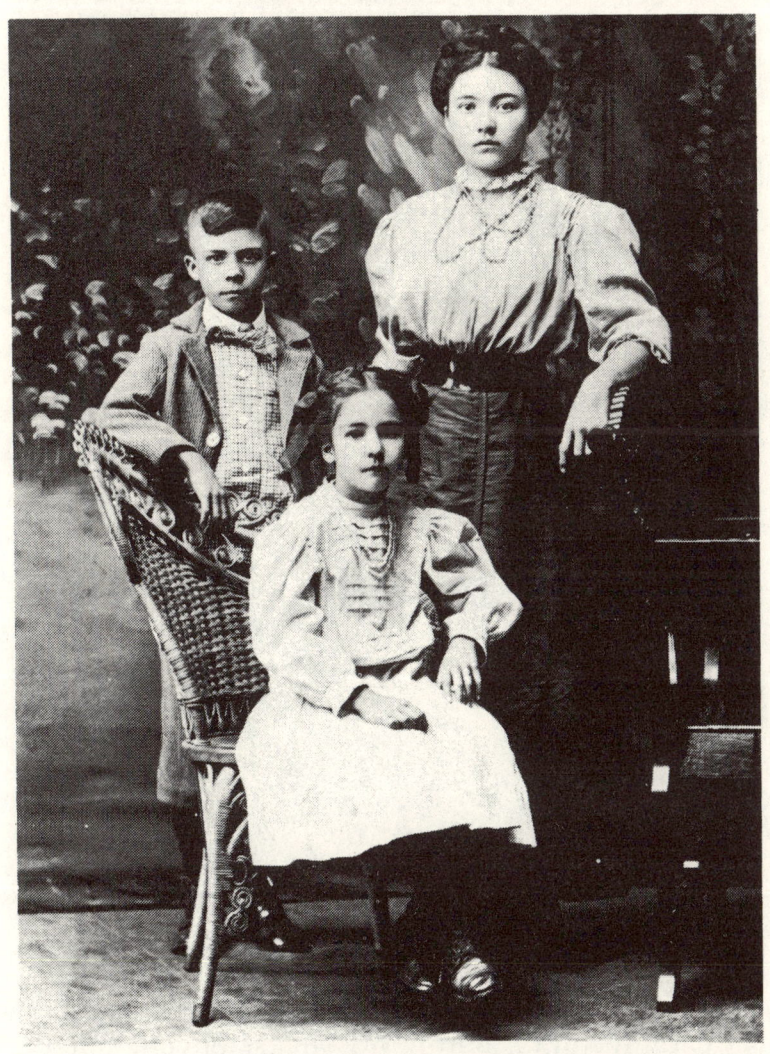

Young Milton with sisters Florence (standing) and Winifred at their family home in Lowell, Wisconsin. Circa 1910.

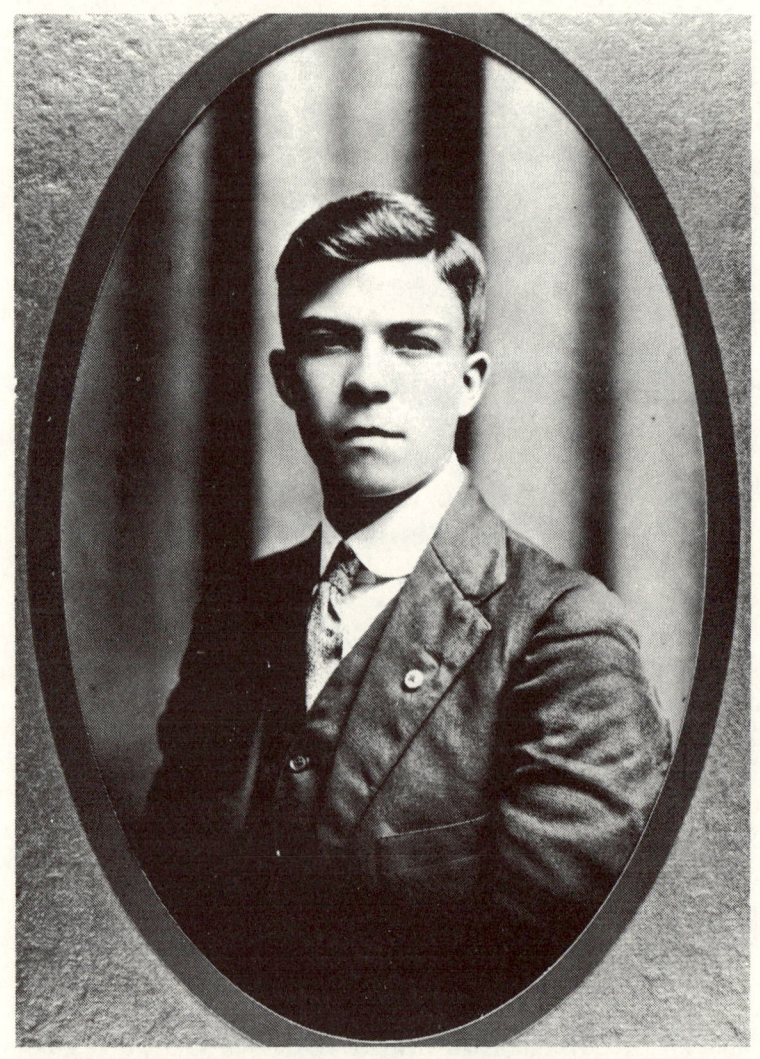

An earnest Milton during his undergraduate college years at the University of Wisconsin. Circa 1922.

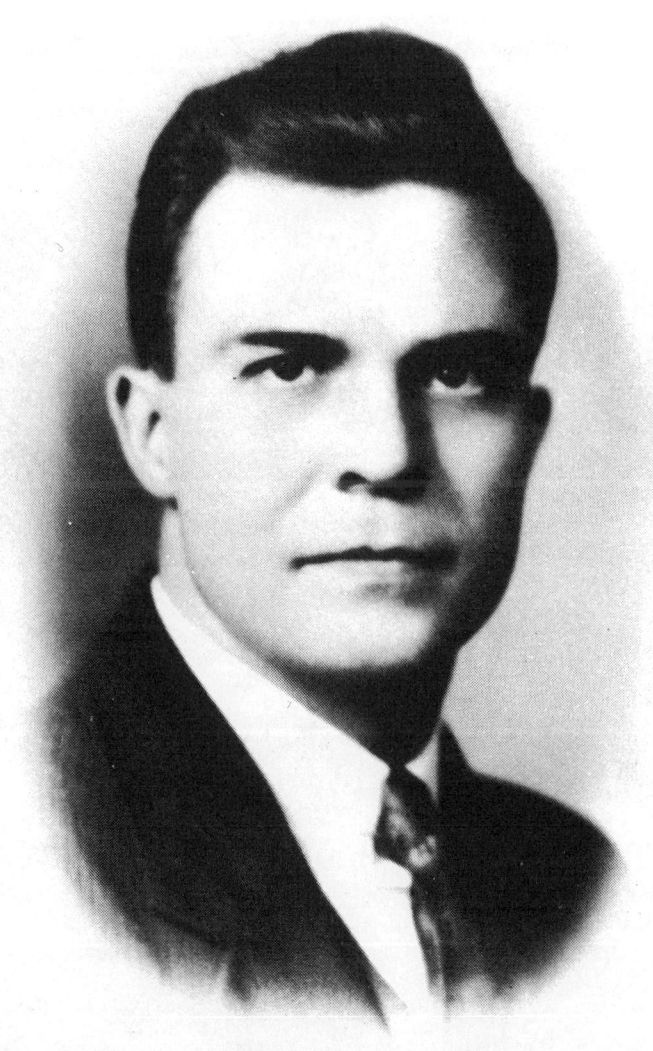

Portrait of Dr. Erickson during his early years of dedicated research at Wayne County General Hospital in Eloise, Michigan. 1938.

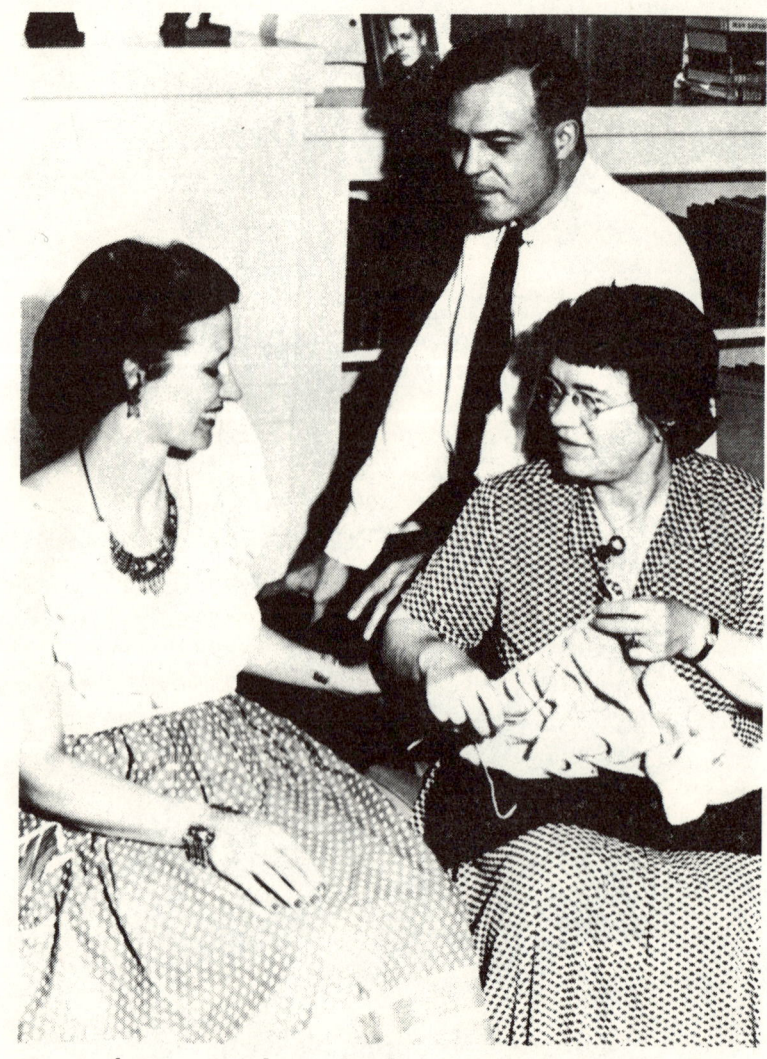

Dr. and Mrs. Erickson in their Phoenix home with a special family friend, Dr. Margaret Mead. June, 1950.

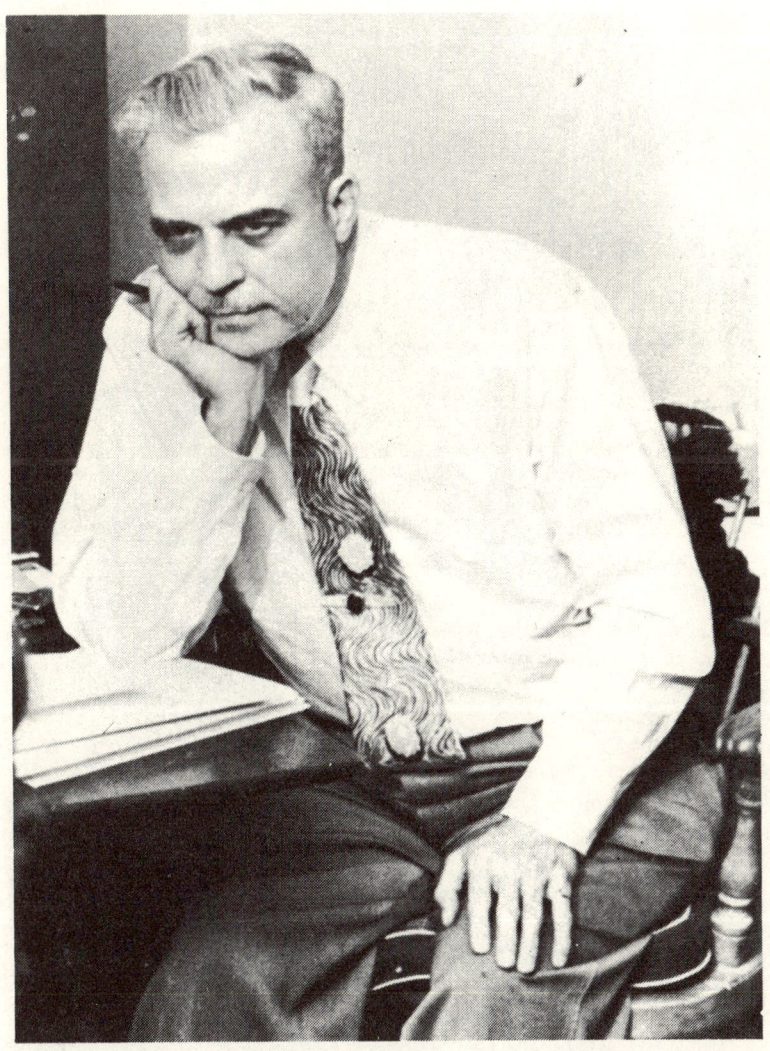

Erickson at work in his home office, a single-pointed focus. 1957.

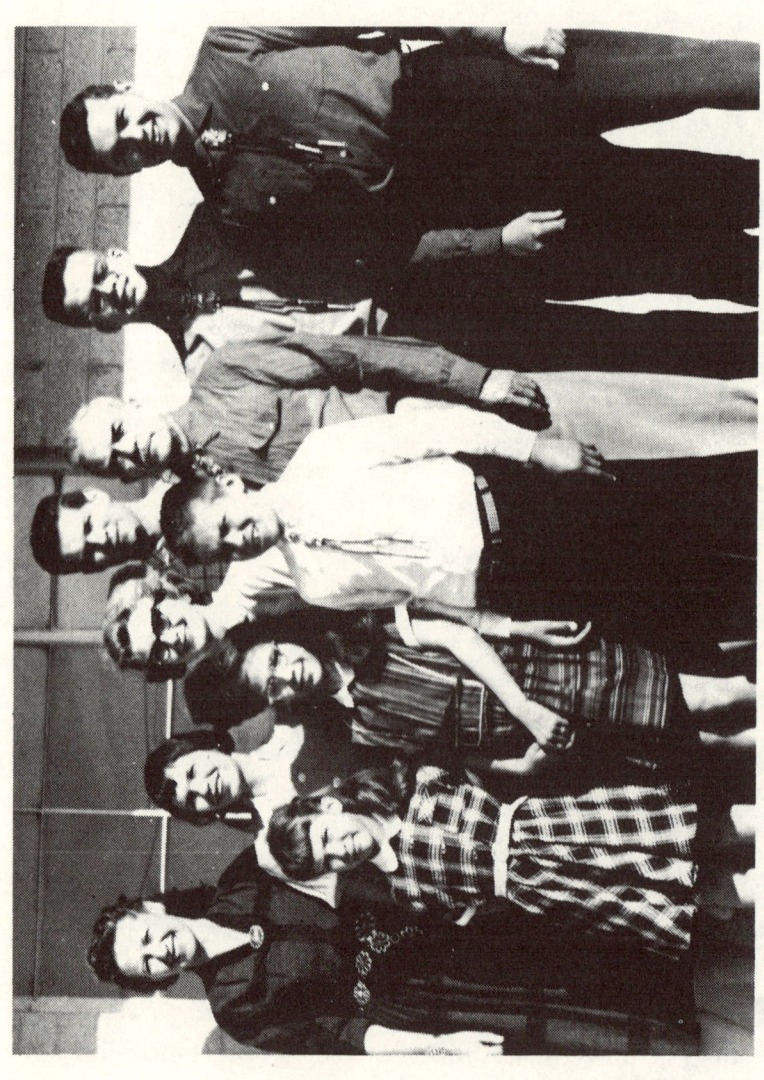

A Thanksgiving family portrait in Phoenix, 1958. One of only two photos of the entire family. Back row (left to right): Mrs. Elizabeth Erickson, Carol, Betty Alice, Lance, Dr. Erickson, Allan, Albert. Front row: Kristina, Roxana, Robert.

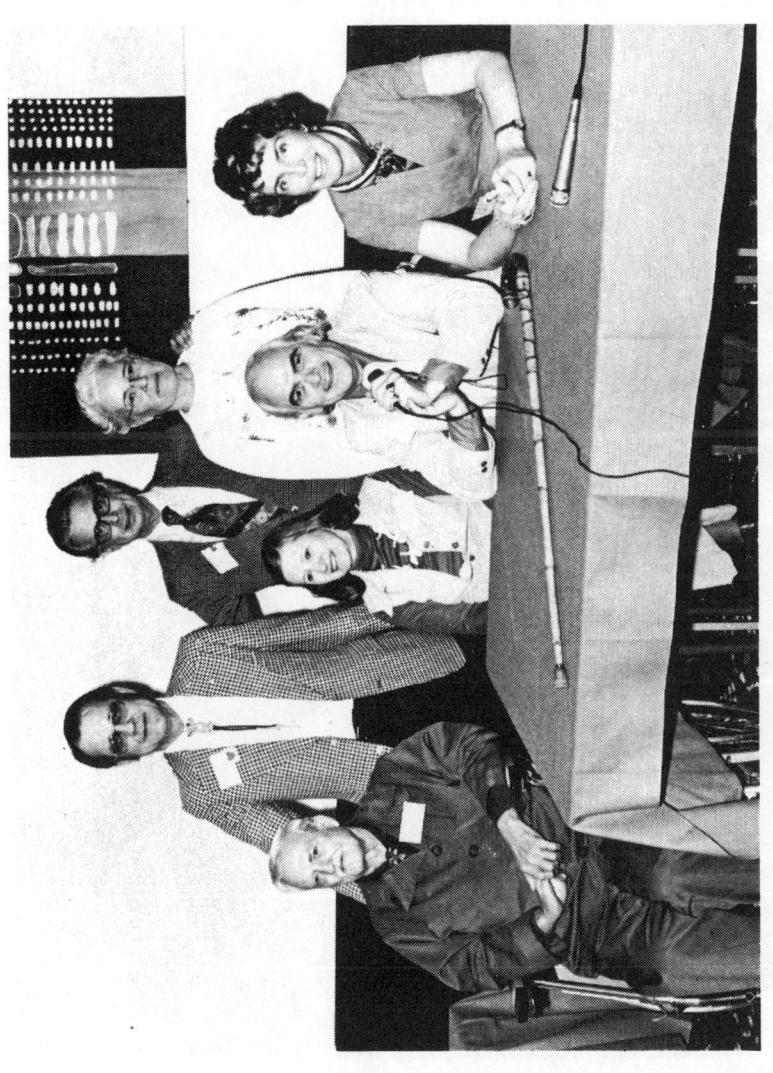

Dr. Erickson with some of his earliest students and collaborators at the 1975 Scientific Meetings of The American Society of Clinical Hypnosis. Standing (left to right): Robert Pearson, Franz Baumann, Bertha Rodgers. Sitting: Dr. Erickson, Mrs. Erickson, Marion Moore, Kay Thompson.

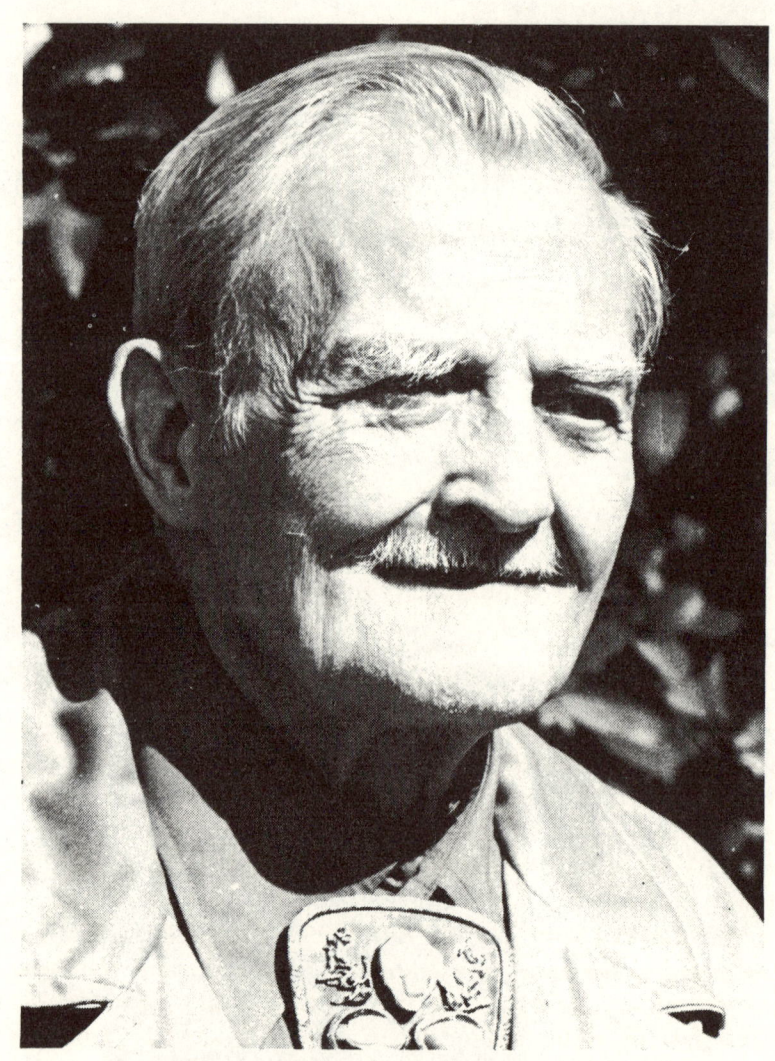

Portrait of a seeker in reflection. Undated.

PART II

REFRAMING PROBLEMS INTO CONSTRUCTIVE ACTIVITY*

Demonstrating Indirect Hypnotic Induction

Reinduction via Revivification of Previous Trance Memories; Open-Ended Suggestions for Future Trance Experience; Age Regression without Asking for It

The presentation this afternoon will concern this matter of indirect induction techniques. And the question is, what constitutes an indirect induction technique? Now, what I think I will do is to begin with an indirect induction technique.

E: [Voice softens into trance tone as Erickson addresses two subjects he hopes but is not sure are present in the audience.] There are in the audience two subjects that I've had in a trance before. One was in one place; one was in another place. And when I put somebody in a trance, I'm very likely to talk about this and I'm very likely to talk about that.

And, for example, I could talk about, let us say, sitting on the shore of the lake; and watching the water, and watching the swimmers, and picking up a stone, and throwing the stone out into the water. A casual conversation. And one could meet a stranger there, and talk to him about this and

*Meeting of The American Society of Clinical Hypnosis in Chicago, Illinois, October 1958.

that, and offer him a package of matches. And will you please come up and sit down in this chair? [Long Pause]

You see, I don't even know if the person is in this room, so I'll try making an approach to the other subject—but I don't know if he is in the room either.

E: [Voice softens] Now, it was at another seminar, and I summarized the presentation of the seminar. And I suggested to you among the others that you go into a trance. And slowly, leisurely, you went into a trance, deeper and deeper and deeper. And everything that I'm saying now applies to a lot of people. And as you went into the trance, you went deeper and deeper, and then you came to my room because of your arm. And now will you slowly stand up and come to the front of the room? [Long pause as the subject, Dr. Bernie Gorton, slowly walks forward.] And will you sit down here, please?

Now all of you heard Dr. Bernie Gorton present to this group, and all of you heard him last night when he presented—at least I hope you did. *Now what is this indirect induction technique? It is simply the process of reminding.*

E: Where are we, Bernie?

B: In Memphis? [They are actually in Chicago.]

E: Yes, we are in Memphis.

You know, I couldn't remember where it was that Dr. Gorton had gone into a trance for me, so I asked Seymour and I asked Pat, and we couldn't figure it out. But it was in Memphis. And yet Dr. Gorton went into a trance when, in speaking to the audience, I asked him to recall a previous trance experience. Now I'm demonstrating this particular induction technique for a very good reason.

E: Bernie, you can put your arm down here on your lap. And enjoy sleeping deeply, and soundly, and restfully. It's been a very nice time in Memphis.

Now and then you will have a patient come to you who says, "I've been hypnotized by someone else, and I'm not certain that I can go into a trance for you." Well, why should you argue or debate that issue? It's false; it's not even pertinent. Therefore you ask the person: "When was it you were hypnotized?... By whom?... How did he do it?... What did he say?... Were you sitting in a chair?... Were you facing a window?... What did you see out the window?... What did the doctor say to you?...

As your patient answers your questions he revives more and more of his memories, and pretty soon he is in the same trance that the other doctor had him in. In other words it is a revival of the original trance, just as Dr. Gorton now revived the original trance of Memphis. He comes up here and he's in Memphis. It's just the revival of the original trance. In that way you can get around a great many difficulties.

Suppose the doctor unwisely tells his patient, "Don't ever let any other doctor hypnotize you—you just be my patient." Now the patient is going to resent that, but he may act on that posthypnotic suggestion and have difficulty going into a trance for you. And as you get more and more experienced, you will find that now and then a patient will say, "I don't know what's wrong with me today, but I have the feeling that you cannot possibly put me in a trance." It may be some silly little whim on his part, but it's true—you can't put him in a trance if you try to do so directly. What do you do? You ask him rather simply and openly: "Now let's see. The last time I put you in a trance was about two weeks ago; you were sitting in this particular chair; we had been conversing about the painting on the wall; and let's see, I suggested hand levitation to you—do you recall that?" You merely reminisce about that previous trance. Once your patient goes into trance you can state quite openly and honestly, "Now, if you want to continue in the trance, you may; but if you want to awaken, it will also be all right. But I would like to have you know that *you can go into a trance any time that you wish, and you can come out of the trance any time that you wish."*

Now, this matter of regression can be brought about this easily. Dr. Gorton is back in Memphis. Trance revivification is a very nice way of securing regression without actually asking somebody to regress.

E: By the way, was I talking to anybody, Bernie? Was I talking to anybody?

B: When?

E: Just now.

B: I think so.

E: It wasn't really important enough to listen, was it? [Long pause] Are you comfortable? And now I would like to have you rouse up and feel rested and refreshed and very, very pleased.

You see, there's nothing difficult about that sort of indirect induction. Any one of you can do it. All I did was talk about something that happened in the past, and we can all reminisce. Now I shall try the other gentleman.

Demonstrating a Second Reinduction

Revivification of Previous Trance Memories; Reorienting the Present into the Future

**E: [Voice softens] Let us sit down on the shore of the lake. The water is as smooth as velvet. Is that a boat out there, or are those people swimming? Are you a stranger here? And let's see this package of matches—what does it read? Hotel Mont Le Mond. Do you smoke? And now slowly will you stand up and come over toward me, slowly, gradually, come over. [Long pause] And that water does look nice out there, doesn't it? [Pause] Don't you wish you could... [inaudible] ... on me? It's a little cold, yes it is. By the way, have I introduced myself?

Subject (S): No.

E: Well, I'd like to meet you, and I don't know if you'd like to meet me. My name is Erickson, and yours?

S: [Gives name.]

E: And how do you happen to be here?

S: We're having a family reunion.

E: Are you having a good time at the family reunion? By the way, you know sometime—I don't know just when, but I think it will be sometime around October, 1958—you're going to meet Dr. Erickson at the Hotel in Chicago. [Pause] And you're going to mention a certain thing to him. And then you're going to get another and very, very comfortable feeling about this matter of going fishing. You don't know what I'm talking about, do you? That is all right. But you'll meet this doctor called Erickson at the Continental Hilton Hotel in October, 1958. I'm sure you will enjoy talking to him. I know that he will enjoy talking to you. And the subject of fishing will come up, and you'll get a new understanding of fishing, [pause] a very enjoyable understanding of fishing. Okay? And everything else will be straightened out too, okay? All right. Now close your eyes and sleep deeply and soundly. That's right, close your eyes. That's right. It's sort of hard to do that for a total stranger, isn't it? But you might as well play along, isn't that right? That's it. And now your hand can go down in your lap—no harm in that—and take a deep breath, and awaken feeling rested and refreshed and energetic. Hi!

S: [Laughs softly.]

E: What's that?

S: You pulled a whiz on me! [Audience laughter]

E: That's what you call the indirect technique! [More laughter]

S: I had a very strange experience. I was in here the first time you talked about matches, and it evoked no memory. I felt strange. And the minute you mentioned the Mont Le Mond Hotel it all came back to me.

E: Then it came back to you—the Mont Le Mond Hotel.

S: How did you remember the name of that hotel? [Laughter]

E: Well, I just keep a vast supply of these little inconsequential things—they come in so handy! [Laughter] Well, thank you very much.

S: You're very welcome.

My very manner of speaking to both subjects compelled them to revivify their memories. I elicited from them responses that could be made only right here, right now. You see, I very seldom go through an elaborate procedure of reorientation when I can do it briefly, quickly, and in a time-saving fashion. And that concludes my presentation of indirect induction techniques.

> Eds: Apparently Erickson had previously hypnotized this subject at the Hotel Mont Le Mond. When the subject says, "And the minute you mentioned the Mont Le Mond Hotel it all came back to me," he is apparently referring back to his previous encounter with Erickson and re-experiencing the subjective sense of that earlier trance.

Similarites between Reinduction and Induction Techniques

There are a couple of comments that I want to make, and Dr. Pattie is responsible for both of them. He pointed out that the demonstration I gave was a demonstration of indirect *re*induction. That is, the patients had been in trances before, and I merely *re*induced them. I chose to make use of people who had been in trances before in order to make it clearer to the audience in this teaching situation. But you can use exactly the same technique on a total stranger by asking him to tell you about some place he has been before, which *you've* never seen. You get him to talk to you about that particular place, and then you can suggest that he sees the water, or the trees, or the flowers, or whatever he looked at when he was at that place.

Making Mistakes

Utilizing Linguistic Errors and Unconscious Corrective Abilities; Splitting Infinitives

Now, the other matter concerns the very nice thing that Dr. Mann did. It was an error so far as words are concerned, but it was not an error so far as teaching is concerned. I expect that Dr. Mann is all ears, wondering what I'm talking about. He said, "*Visualize* a breeze." Too often we become overly concerned about our errors. For heaven's sake, never take the attitude that you can't make mistakes in working with patients. Sometimes an important consideration in a hypnotic technique can come about through an error in language.

I recall a Smith College student who pointed out to me that I split infinitives. Her father was a professor of English—you just didn't split infinitives in that family! But once this question of split infinitives came up, she got very interested in explaining to me how I was ruining my technique, and how she could respond easily if only I would just quit splitting those infinitives. And she called my attention to each one. After that interaction I realized that I *ought* to use split infinitives because she couldn't stand to hear them and she would go into a trance just to avoid listening to me! [Laughter] She had a doctorate in psychology, so we discussed her reactions later.

The point is that you must realize you can make mistakes; you don't have to be apologetic, and you can go right on. The unconscious mind is intelligent, and it will recognize that you don't *visualize* a breeze, and therefore you get the patient's unconscious to participate by automatically correcting your little error.

Learning to Verbalize

Now, I have one final comment on Dr. Mann's presentation, which impressed me very much. I would like to have you consider the importance of learning how to verbalize as a beginning experience, so that you can learn to utilize your own capacity to observe and to talk to a patient simply. Dr. Mann said, "Relax the muscles of your face; relax the muscles around your mouth; relax the muscles around your jaw." In other words, he repeated the same thing in three different and very simple ways. You can always say the same thing in different ways, and you need never be at a loss for something to say. The important consideration is your willingness to accept the patient's behavior as good.

Hypnosis as Cooperation

Developing Hypnotic Techniques in Relation to the Free Expression of Patient and Therapist Personalities; the Need for Skill and Judgment

In presenting this seminar as an advanced seminar on hypnosis, we wish to extend some of the benefit of our experience, of our teaching, of our own trade. We would like to try to give you some new understandings that we do not cover in the beginning seminars.

One of the matters I've taken up from time to time with the

advanced group has been this question of hypnotic techniques. We've been very careful to try to teach you different methods of inducing trances. We feel that it is very important for you to know as many different techniques as possible, for the only way you can develop your own technique is by an awareness of all the different techniques—whether it's the house-tree-man technique, the coin technique, the relaxation technique, or whatever it happens to be. You see, *hypnosis is a matter of cooperation between the patient and yourself. The only way you can secure that cooperation is when a patient is free to express his own personality, and when you are free to express your own personality.*

Each of you has different aspects to your personality: you react to one person in one way, and you react to another person in a different way. Because you react to different personalities in different ways, you ought to have techniques that express each aspect of your personality. You'll encounter patients who demand of you a domineering technique, so you ought to be acquainted with that type of technique as *you* would express it—not as you would copy it from someone else. Therefore you should be acquainted with all the various techniques, and you should want to practice them. All of these techniques take a bit of time to learn how to use, and you are all busy people. You haven't got too much time to devote to each individual patient. As beginners you need to hypnotize—or to try to hypnotize—as many of your patients as possible. You need to do that for two reasons: one reason is to discover how to recognize those patients you cannot hypnotize, and the other is to discover how to recognize those patients you do not need to hypnotize.

Hypnosis as Responding to Ideas

A Hand Levitation Technique Evoking Wonder, Doubt, and Inner Search to Facilitate Relaxation and Receptivity: "What Does He Want My Hand to Do?"

I can think of some more discoveries you can use in order to develop skill. One of my dental friends told me that when he first started using hypnosis, he put every patient who came into his office into a trance—or else he tried very hard to put every patient into a trance! Now he has discovered a change in his approach: he simply looks at his patients and addresses a few words to them in order to decide whether or not hypnosis is warranted or indicated.

He made another very nice discovery, which is the matter I want to bring to your attention today. He doesn't attempt to relax his patients, and he doesn't attempt the coin technique. He has a patient sit down in a chair, and then he asks if he can place the patient's arm on the armrest of the chair. That is, may he take hold of the patient's hand, take hold of the patient's wrist, and very carefully lay it on the arm of the chair? In so doing, he moves the patient's hand up and down like this, while addressing simple, casual remarks to the patient. What he is really doing is asking the patient's permission to manipulate the arm, and then he proceeds to manipulate the arm.

What is the point? The patient cannot see any particular reason for such an action, any particular purpose in it, and so *he wonders and speculates and is literally wide open for the presentation of an idea.* What you want your patient to do in hypnosis is to respond to an idea. And it is your task, your responsibility, to learn how to address the patient; how to speak to the patient; how to secure the patient's attention; how to leave the patient wide open to the acceptance of an idea that fits into the situation.

When my friend takes hold of his patient's wrist and starts moving it slowly up and down, the patient wonders to himself, *Is he testing me for relaxation, or is he trying to fit my hand over the end of the arm of the chair? What does he want my hand to do?* And as the patient begins that sort of thinking—*What does he want my hand to do?*—the dentist then can say, "And just continue relaxing more and more." This technique takes about 10 to 30 seconds. In that moment of inner inquiry—*What does he want my hand to do?* —the patient is completely ready to accept whatever idea is presented to him. He then receives the reply, "Just relax more and more."

All of you have seen me take hold of a volunteer's wrist, lift the arm, and suggest that he go into a deep trance. That is exactly the same sort of technique as this dentist uses. I do it in front of a group because I want to demonstrate hypnosis as a deep phenomenon rather rapidly. But your willingness to attract attention and to allow the patient to be in mental doubt as to what he should think and what he should do in that particular situation makes him amenable to any suggestion you give him (provided it fits that immediate situation). You see, *hypnosis doesn't come from mere repetition. It comes from getting your patient to accept an idea and to respond to that idea.* It doesn't have to be a wealth of ideas. It can be one single idea presented at the opportune moment so that the patient can give his full attention to it. In dealing with patients, your entire purpose is to secure their attention, to secure their cooperation, and to make certain that they respond.

Explaining the Conscious-Unconscious Minds

Listening With The Unconscious; Irrelevance of Conscious Mental Activity; the Conscious-Unconscious Double Bind

Another consideration I want to emphasize to you is the following. Too often the beginning practitioner in hypnosis makes an effort to lullabye the conscious mind by constant repetitious suggestions; to tell the patient that he is tired, that he is going to sleep, that he is relaxing more and more. Instead, the beginning operator needs to recognize that *his primary task is that of addressing himself to the patient: the patient's attention must be arrested sufficiently so that he can listen with his unconscious mind.* I think it is much more important to tell a patient that he knows, as you know, that there is the "front" of his mind, that there is the "back" of his mind; that there is the "conscious" mind, that there is the "unconscious" mind. He needs to be told that he can listen with his conscious mind while his unconscious mind is busy with a wealth of other things; that it is perfectly possible to listen with the unconscious mind while the conscious mind is occupied with other things. You need to explain to most patients that they do not know what the unconscious mind is doing, or what it is going to do, or what it is going to think; and that *no matter what the conscious mind is thinking or doing, the unconscious mind can carry on its own independent activity. It does not take very long to explain that to patients, and then you tell them that you would like them to listen to you with the conscious mind if they wish, but primarily you would like to have them listen with their unconscious mind—a response of which they will not be aware.*[1]

Separating the Conscious and Unconscious

Associating a Suggestion with a Behavioral Inevitability; Tailoring Unconscious Learnings to Individual Needs and Capacities

Now I know that this sounds as if I am establishing a psychological dichotomy, treating the mind as if it were comprised of two separate entities. In function, the unconscious and conscious minds often are separate entities. I tell my patients that they really do not need to listen to me with their conscious minds. My objective is to make it apparent that they do not need to fix their attention on me laboriously. They can let the conscious mind wander at will—and the conscious mind *does* wander at will—but in so speaking to them, I am literally giving them an instruction and a suggestion about what they are going to do. They are going to do it anyway, but since I mention it they will be doing it in response to my suggestion. *And if they let their conscious minds wander, having accepted that suggestion, then they feel obligated to listen to me with their unconscious minds, since I have also mentioned that.*[2]

I explain to patients that as they listen to me with their unconscious minds, they can learn all of the things that they need to learn. They do not need to be consciously aware of what they are learning; that, in fact, they have the privilege of using what they learn unconsciously at the time and at the place best fitted to their own needs. Patients need to be reassured that what happens to them is going to be in accord with their actual needs and with their actual capacities. Too many patients come into the office with the feeling that the therapist must overpower them, or that he must drive home a wealth of ideas at a conscious level. I want to avoid that particular approach because I like to work rapidly, and I do not like to waste my time on repetitious suggestions of every sort. When I first started using hypnosis I worked out very, very elaborate and extensive techniques of suggestions of every sort. But the more experience I've had, the more I have cut down on the number of those suggestions.

Hypnosis Without Awareness of It

Focusing on Hypnotic Purpose Rather Than Hypnotic Depth

Now, another general matter that I want to impress upon you concerns awareness. Is it really necessary for your patient to know that he is hypnotized? Does it serve any good purpose for either you or your patient to know that you put him in a trance? What does the patient really need? He primarily needs the responsiveness and the receptiveness of the hypnotic state. He doesn't need to *know* that he is in the trance state; he is there for medical or dental reasons, for reasons other than the experience of being hypnotized. In a teaching situation your patient might want to know that he was in the hypnotic state, but the patient who comes to you for medical or dental aid is not interested in knowing that he is in a light trance or a medium trance or a deep trance, or half-way in between. It serves no real purpose because he is there, perhaps, to have some sutures taken out.

Another example is the child who comes to you to have a laceration sewed up. Is it important for him to know that he is in a trance—that he is in a light trance or a medium trance or a deep trance? The essential thing for the child to know is that he can enjoy having that laceration sutured. The idea must be presented in such a way that it sounds like a completely, perfectly delightful thing to the child. You do not need a trance state that is recognized by the child, so that he can say, for instance,

"Yes, I am in a trance; I am deep asleep." All that child needs to know is that he is going to have suturing done, that he is going to see the needle go in and out; he is going to watch and see what mother is doing, what the doctor is doing, what the nurse is doing. He just needs to be interested in the total situation. He does not need to be interested in knowing: "Am I in a trance?... Am I going to go deeper in the trance?... Am I cataleptic? ... Am I unaware of my surroundings? ... Am I paying attention to this one thing or paying attention to a wealth of other things?"

Too often in medical and dental practice the effort is made to get the patient to recognize too much about the trance state. Too much effort is made to direct his critical faculties toward ascertaining the *degree* of the hypnosis rather than directing his interest to the accomplishment of the *purposes* of the hypnosis. Your hypnosis should be oriented around the task to be accomplished. It should not be oriented around a recognition of one psychological state or another.

Redirecting the Subject's Attention

Hypnosis as a Process of Distraction, Fixation, and Generalization

Now, how does one handle that sort of thing? Do you do it by repetitious suggestion? Do you do it by distracting your patient's attention? Or do you do it by fixating the patient's attention? I think you ought to bear in mind that your awareness of hypnosis should make you keenly appreciative of the significance of fixation and the significance of distraction.

The nurse untrained in hypnosis confronted by a patient who says, "I always faint when I get a hypodermic injection," can very easily pinch the skin over that patient's deltoid or the triceps and say in return: "I wonder if I should give you the hypodermic injection here, or here? Well, there's the syringe over there, but let me first feel your deltoid and your triceps."

The patient knows that his deltoid is being felt, that his triceps are being felt, and he is giving his attention to the feeling of having those muscles felt. And so the nurse has distracted the patient's attention entirely to this matter of the sensation of her fingers on the skin, pressing the tissue. And eventually she picks up a syringe out of the patient's sight, and gives the hypodermic injection while the patient's attention is fixated on the pinch. Of course, the patient is watching another syringe "over there" which he thought she was going to use: a distraction—a bald, obvious distraction technique.

But what is the entire purpose of the visit to the office? Is it to explain to the patient: "I will now squeeze on the tissue"; "I will now pick up the syringe"; "I will now plunge the needle into the skin"? That serves no legitimate purpose in increasing either the patient's understanding or his cooperation. The patient knows you are going to give him a hypodermic injection. The patient comes for that purpose. That's all the cooperation you need in order to plunge the hypodermic needle into the tissue.

The other cooperation you need is the cooperation that allows the patient to gaze on that syringe "over there" (that is not actually used) and to focus attention on the feeling of the nurse's fingers on his tissues "right here." That's all the cooperation that the patient can give you for the hypodermic injection. You need to employ distraction. You need to explain the situation in some indirect way, by act or comment or by the raising of a question. You need to direct the patient's attention toward the particular things that he needs to do in order to accomplish the purposes for which he came.

What is the dentist doing when he takes hold of the hand and wrist of his patient; when he puts the patient's arm on the armrest of the chair so that it will be nicely relaxed? He is distracting the patient's attention from his neck, from his face, from his body, from his legs. He is getting the patient to comprehend what relaxation is. As soon as the patient shows relaxation in the arm, wrist, and hand—thereby discovering what relaxation is—the dentist can generalize it by saying, "Now relax all over." The patient is already giving his full attention to relaxation. You merely ask him to spread the relaxation which he is experiencing in his arm and wrist and hand to the rest of his body. In other words, the dentist first distracts the patient's attention from the mouth, re-focuses the attention on the sensation of relaxation, and then generalizes this relaxation over the entire body, including the mouth.

Hypnosis as Receiving and Responding to Ideas

Fixating the Patient on Ideas Evoking Wonder and Questioning: Utilizing the Need for Answers

Now the question is, Is that hypnosis? Primarily, *hypnosis is a matter of getting the patient to be receptive to ideas and to respond to ideas*. There are various ways of getting the patient to respond to ideas. One is to hammer home the idea until, in desperation, the patient gives his attention to it; another is to present the idea to him in such a gentle, appealing way that you arouse his interest immediately and completely.

The other aspect of "attention getting" lies in the area of fixation. One can distract the patient and direct the attention indirectly to this or that particular thing. But one can also go about it in another way. In teaching you the relaxation technique, Aston has demonstrated the importance of looking at a spot on the ceiling or on the wall. In the coin technique, you look at the thumbnail and you fix your attention on the movement of the fingers. There are various ways of fixating the attention. For beginners, for those just learning, you need practice. You need to have some fixation spot of attention: a particular spot on the wall, your thumbnail, a bright, shiny thing, the sensation of your hands resting on your thighs, the feeling of a coin resting in your hand, a visual image in your mind's eye.

There are many ways of getting a fixation, but what is the *best* way of getting a fixation? The best way is *not* to rely on external reality or on a visual image of external reality. Rather, *get the patient to fixate on an idea or a thought that is unformu-*

lated. Now you saw that rather elaborate gesture. [Erickson moves a pencil about in the air.] Did it serve any particular purpose? [He gestures in the same way again.] All that the patient can do when you act in that way is to wonder, "Now what is the meaning of that? What explanation can there be for that kind of movement? Is the doctor puzzled about his pencil? Does he want it in any particular position on the desk? Just exactly what is the meaning of all this?" And it does look as if there must be a meaning, a value. *The patient is what I call "wide open" to the reception of some idea about that pencil. He wants information.* You have deliberately, intentionally fixated attention on the pencil; Then you look at the pencil again, and then you move it over here, over there, and the patient is obliged to follow the movement of that pencil.

Fixating Attention With Children

Utilizing Distraction and Wonder

The patient that you use that technique on most effectively is the small child. The small child who comes into your office, doesn't like your white coat, doesn't like the pictures on your walls, doesn't like anything about the situation. He does not like the possibility that you might give him "shots." He just doesn't like anything. Now what do you do about that child?

You have a hunting case watch. You snap open the case thoughtfully and you look at the time thoughtfully. You close it, and you open it again. You are fixing the child's gaze on that watch. Take the watch off your wrist and lay it down here; move it to there. The child is probably thinking, "I am glad he is thinking about that watch and not giving me shots!"

That is what I want to accomplish: get the child thinking about the watch, get his thoughts away from himself and his own thinking, get him thinking about the thing that I present to him, and get him to fixate his gaze on a focal point so that he gives his full attention to that one focal point. Then I am in a position to ask him to think about the conscious mind and the unconscious mind; and then a word to suggest to him that he give his attention in the manner that I request.

Successful Hypnosis in Medical Settings

Focusing Attention away from Unpleasant External Realities and onto Beneficient Inner Processes

As soon as I have secured the patient's attention and maneuvered it around a bit, I can ask him to notice the difference in the weight of his thumb and his little finger as each rests on his thigh. And the patient gives his attention to that, because it does apply to him. Now, do I want the patient to fixate his attention on external realities: on my watch, on the paperweight on the desk, on the spot on the wall; or, do I want him to attend to his own inner experiential happenings, to his own psychosomatic processes and sensations? I want the patient's attention directed within himself. I want him to fixate his attention on the processes taking place within him. *Whether you are practicing psychiatry, dermatology, obstetrics, or dentistry, you need to get the patient to pay attention to the processes within himself, rather than to thoughts about what you are going to do to him externally.*

What are those processes within him that he needs to pay attention to? Do you want him to pay attention to the needle that you are going to shove into him in suturing his wound? No. That is what you will be doing to him externally. Instead, you want him to pay attention to the goodness and the niceness of the full expectation that his body will become well and unwounded again.

What is it that you want of the obstetrical patient? Do you want her to have the feeling that she must tell the nurse that she's having another pain? Do you want her to give her attention to the pain of labor contractions, or to the feeling of movement within her own body? Do you want her to have the feeling of gripping the handgrips in pain, or the feeling of a muscle contraction in her forearm? You want her to fixate her attention where it's going to do her the greatest amount of good. You don't want her attention directed in any way to externalities that are going to disturb or distress her. In the functioning of the human body there are a sufficient number of good processes, of pleasing processes, no matter what is going on, for the patient to attend to. You want to distract patients away from the unpleasant goings-on, and re-direct them to the desirable, beneficent processes that will aid them in cooperating with you.

Temporal Considerations in Hypnosis

Establishing Appropriate Time Requirements via a "Triple-Layered Recognition" of the Patient: Person, Patient, and Problem

Now another consideration in this matter of hypnosis is your appreciation of time value. Too often you have the feeling that hypnosis must be a time consuming proposition, and the tone of your voice, the way you look at your patient, the way you start speaking, your reaction to the clock on your desk—all indicate that you expect to take a certain amount of time. Instead, you ought to give the patient the feeling that you will give him all the time that he wants, all the time that he needs, and all the time that is necessary.

First let me explain the phrase, "all the time that he wants." He doesn't want you to rush your time. He wants you to take your time. It has nothing to do with him. It's your time and he is paying you for it, and he wants you to take plenty of it. Next you shift the focus onto the time that he needs. Now how much time does he need? He doesn't need *all* of your time. There is already an understanding of that fact in his mind. It turns out he only wants *part* of your time, a small amount of your time. And so you shift from all the time he *wants* to all the time he *needs;* but it's what *he* needs, he, as a person, as a patient—all the time that *he needs*.

Now that brings us to how much time is necessary? You have reduced the requirement from all of the doctor's time and all the time the patient needs to the time that is necessary for the particular procedure for which the patient comes to you. And gently, unobtrusively, you have reduced the time requirements to whatever time is necessary for actual office procedures, and nothing more. In that way, you have transformed the total situation from one of one person meeting another person, into one of a patient meeting a professional person, into one of a problem being dealt with by both. And that is the orientation that you should provide.

But first you do go through the process. Initially you do have the orientation of another person dealing with you as a professional person; then you have the orientation of dealing with your patient as a person, a sick person; then you gain a refined recognition of the specific problem of this patient, who has come to you as a fellow citizen. And so you've got a triple-layered recognition of your patient: one as a person, one as a patient, and one as a presenting problem. The clarity with which you recognize each of these aspects helps to cut down the length of time for the visit, and allows you to give the patient an understanding that your allotment of time will be the correct, the desired, the appropriate length of time.

Directing Ideas to the Unconscious Mind

Enlisting Attention and Evoking Response Readiness via Arm Levitation: Confusion and Lack of Understanding Facilitating Response Readiness

When you try to combine a fixation and distraction of attention in addition to this utilization of talking to the unconscious mind, you need not be harried by a fear that maybe the patient's conscious mind is still listening. You can safely assume that the patient's unconscious mind is listening, and that all you need to do is give the patient the opportunity to receive ideas and to respond to them. You become less and less concerned with the need of eliminating the conscious mind. You become less and less concerned with taking time to eliminate the conscious mind, because eliminating the attention of the conscious mind is a time-consuming process. Your time is better spent in enlisting the attention of the unconscious mind. That's why I like to use some such attention focusing procedure as the gentle lifting of an arm. Nobody knows exactly what I mean by such an action. There is no previous experience, learning, or understanding of what I am doing. *This lack of understanding leads to that open readiness to respond.* In such a situation the unconscious is going to be decidedly attentive.

VOCAL DYNAMICS

Fixating Attention and Facilitating Responsiveness

A consideration in this matter of approaching patients is the forcefulness with which you address them. Too often the effort is made to secure the patient's attention by a frontal assault: You tell him he is getting "more and more tired" ... "more and more tired" ... sleepier and sleepier," and so on. That's a rather forceful way of doing it. Now how many of you have talked to deaf people who, in reaction to their own deafness, speak in practically subliminal tones so that you have to strain to hear them? In this matter of getting your patient's attention you ought to talk to him in such a fashion that you keep him *right on the edge of attentiveness.* You do not talk too loudly; neither do you talk in too low a tone. You try to talk to him as if you were speaking just *to him,* and not including this water pitcher. Your voice is only going to carry from you to the patient, right here, and no further. You need to understand that, and to analyze your own reaction to that particular way of addressing a patient. It keeps the patient fixing his attention on you. You never talk in too low a tone of voice because it tires out your patient. You never make him strain unduly. You just ask the minimum effort from him so that all of his energy is given to an acceptance and an understanding and a responsiveness to ideas.

Distracting Consciousness

*Hand Levitation and Catalepsy Approaches: Tactile Cues
Suggesting an Upward Movement*

Now, I can illustrate this point in another manner. I think all of you have seen me take hold of a patient's arm, lift it up and move it about in various ways, thereby inducing a trance. And I've tried to teach a number of you how to take hold of a wrist, how to take hold of a hand. You do not grip with all the strength in your hand and squeeze down on the wrist. What you do is take hold of it very, very gently and suggest the grip of the wrist. But you don't really grip it: you suggest a movement of the wrist; you suggest a movement of the hand; you suggest an upward movement. How do you suggest an upward movement? You press here on the thumb, just slightly, while at the same time you're moving this finger this way to give it balance. You're moving your finger this way laterally, and the patient gives attention to that thumb lifting the hand, or to that thumb *suggesting* the lifting of the hand.

Now what happens is that the patient unwittingly tends to follow out your suggestions by virtue of his consciously directed attention to the firm pressure on the top of his hand, and by virtue of his unconsciously directed attention to the touch of your thumb underneath his hand. That gentle touch indicates that it should remain a gentle touch, and the firm touch is up here. The only way you can get the firm touch to remain firm is to keep moving the hand up against it, and the only way you can keep the lower touch of the thumb on the hand a gentle touch is to keep moving the hand away from it. And so you're suggesting an upward movement against the firm touch to maintain the firm touch; and you're suggesting an upward movement of the hand with the gentle touch by moving the hand up so that it remains a gentle touch. And you need to practice this technique over and over again. *It is one of the quickest and easiest ways of distracting the conscious attention and securing the attention of the unconscious mind.* I think that you ought to practice taking hold of a wrist or a hand at every opportunity.[3]

Extending Unconscious Aid Somatically

Utilizing Tactile Suggestions for Catalepsy as a Pain Distraction Technique; Extending Catalepsy and Anesthesia Throughout the Body

Now how do you suggest catalepsy in that fashion? You lift the hand up in that fashion. Now when does my thumb come away from his thumb? I let it linger there and linger there, so that there will be a sense of *lingering*. Or I draw my hand out this way in such a manner that the patient has a nice, comfortable feeling of the lingering of my hand. You want the patient's attention on his hand. You want the development of that state of muscle tonus, because *once the muscle tonus is established to achieve catalepsy, that means you have enlisted the aid of the unconscious mind throughout all of the patient's body*. If you can get a catalepsy in one hand, there is a good possibility that you can get catalepsy in the other hand. And if you get catalepsy in the other hand, then you've probably got catalepsy in the right foot, and in the left foot, and throughout the body, the face and the neck. And as soon as you get a catalepsy with that balanced tonicity of the muscles you have a physical state that allows the patient to become unaware of any disturbing sensations. It's awfully hard to maintain that balanced muscle tonus and at the same time pay attention to pain. You want your patient giving all of his attention to that muscle tonus.

That is one reason why you need Saturday afternoon sessions. I demonstrated the phenomena of the deep trance so extensively for the purpose of making you realize a wealth of hypnotic phenomena. If you can get muscle tonus and catalepsy in the right arm then you're going to get it in the left arm; you're going to get muscle tonus throughout the body. You've got muscle tonus throughout the body, catalepsy throughout the body; you have reduced the sensations that exist within the body to those sensations that go into maintaining that catalepsy. And the patient becomes decidedly responsive to a wealth of other ideas. If I were to produce an obstetrical anesthesia, one of the things I'd want to teach my patient would be this matter of muscle tonus, this matter of catalepsy. I would want her to feel the catalepsy in her arm or her hand, or to feel it in her face and eyelids, and then I would direct her attention to other sensations in her body at my request. These sensations belong to her, and I can single out the ones that she ought to pay attention to. The more acquainted you are with a variety of hypnotic phenomena, the more easily you can direct the patient.

Pain Control in Hypnosis

Utilizing the Interrelationship of Psychological and Mental Mechanisms: Teaching Amnesia for Pain Via Distraction and the Use of Unrelated, Everyday Examples

Now for muscle tonus. You do not know if your patient can develop an anesthesia. You need to have an understanding that all psychological phenomena are interrelated and that there are a variety of ways of activating them.

I've discussed this matter of anesthesia in a couple of advanced courses. How does one proceed to develop an anesthesia for a patient dying from a painful cancer? You know you can go to a show, a suspense movie, and forget about your toothache. You can go to a suspense movie and forget about your headache. You can have a very pleasant surprise and forget about your aching corn. Therefore, why should you think about pain as necessarily being treated by anesthesia, as necessarily being treated by analgesia? You've all had the experience of forgetting a hurt, which means that you can treat pain by inducing amnesia. You can treat pain by distraction. And that's what you need to recognize in the dental and medical use of hypnosis: *the utilization of the various functions of the human mind in achieving any particular goal.*

When you have an amnesia for pain, what exactly does it do for the pain? Let's take that cancer patient. This man had recurrent, short, stabbing, lancinating bouts of pain, excruciating in character, that occurred about every ten minutes. What was that pain experience—the experience of the pain itself? It was a genuine thing. It included all the psychological reflexes of pain. In addition the patient knew that in another ten minutes he would get another stab of pain. He also knew that ten minutes ago he had had a pain. He also knew that one minute... two minutes... three... four... five minutes had passed, and now it's time for another pain. And so two-thirds of his pain was made up of remembering the last pain, a horrible experience, and anticipating the pain as a coming experience. The remaining third was experiencing the actual bout of pain.

One of the things I did for this man was the simple process of teaching him amnesia, but I taught him amnesia for some simple thing because in medical and dental hypnosis you do not drive home to the core of the problem immediately. When you do an abdominal examination for appendicitis, you do not, when palpitating the abdomen, come right down on the tender spot. You get over to the other side of the abdomen and you move by degrees to where you think the pain is. You examine a painful back in the same way. You try to approach the painful area gently, slowly, carefully, so that you can actually define it instead of sensitizing the entire area by jabbing right down on the painful area.

Psychologically you approach a patient in that same way. You approach the development of an amnesia by telling him: "I would like to have you remember this simple little thing. I'm going to give you four digits. Do you mind remembering the four digits, 4... 7... 81?"

What have you done? You have said, "... four digits, 4... 7... 81." And the patient has to stop and analyze the 81 as 8 and 1. You have named four digits, right? You've made him pause and put all of his attention, not on the 4 and the 7, but on the 8 and the 1. And so he's giving the major part of his attention to the 81.

Then you apologize, "I should have said '8 and 1' instead of '81.'" And the patient accepts your apology.

Then you ask, "Now, what were the other two numbers?" Because the patient is giving so much of his attention to the 81 he tends to forget the 4 and the 7. You've mentioned these last two digits coupled together so frequently that he's forgotten the

157

4 and the 7. You have taught him to fixate his attention. You have taught him to separate his attention. You have taught him to accept an idea; you have taught him to fixate his attention from all other parts of the task. Then you can compliment him upon the fact that he developed an amnesia so quickly, so easily.

How does one develop an amnesia? It's so easily done. You can be introduced to half a dozen people very rapidly. When the introductions are completed you wonder who was who, and what was the first person's name; and while you're trying to figure that out, you're busy forgetting the second person's name; and once you become aware of the second person's name you wonder, "Now, what was the third person's name?" You wind up wishing that the person who had introduced you had taken his time. But it's a very nice way of developing amnesia.

Pain Control in Hypnosis

Utilizing Time Distortion, Individual Time Values, and the Negative to Alter Subjective Experience: Shortening the Pain and Lengthening the Pleasure

In medical and dental hypnosis you first get your patient to accept ideas at a very, very simple level, and then you move on. I taught this man with cancer the importance of forgetting; he could have an amnesia for his lancinating pain. That meant that he could not look forward to having the pain, he could not look backward to having experienced the pain already. Each recurring, lancinating pain was a totally new, surprising experience.

Now how long does a pain last? If you are giving all of your attention to it, it lasts a long time. You have a throbbing toothache, and the more you pay attention to it each throb seems to be a great, long, slow throb. In other words, the time value of the pain becomes tremendously increased and you must be willing to teach a patient (medical or dental) the importance of decreasing that time.

I made this cancer patient understand that the pain would be of very short duration, and I asked him to fix his attention on the expectation that the pain would be so brief that *he might miss it.* A nice idea. But I also encouraged him to feel the pain by fixing his attention on it because *he might miss it,* because it was so brief. My desire was for him to miss the pain. The patient knew that he couldn't miss the pain, but I presented the idea in a negative fashion: he must fix his attention on the pain because it might be so brief that in a moment's inattention *he might miss it.* The effect of this was to convince the patient that his pain was, indeed, short.

> Eds: Note that Erickson's subtle use of the word *might* also indirectly converts the patient's expectation of pain as a *certainty* to pain as a mere *possibility*.

In whatever dental or medical procedure you undertake, you need to recognize the time values of that experience for the patient. You do not want the patient to have a prolonged, unpleasant experience. Therefore, in whatever fashion you can, present the ideas to them that will facilitate the shortening of the subjective time value of that unpleasant experience. You ask the child to see how *fast* the needle goes through the skin in suturing the wound. You want him to notice how *fast* it goes through. He should really pay attention because *he might miss it.* And so you have keyed him to an experience that is going to be very, very fast.

Take the magician who tells you that the hand is faster than the eye, and having told you that, very convincingly proceeds to demonstrate that the hand is faster than the eye. But he has already keyed you to expect that hand to move very rapidly. Key yourself to watch the slowness and gracefulness of that hand moving. He'll be very careful not to move it too fast, because that's what you're expecting. He moves it much more slowly than you anticipate, and your eyes are jumping ahead of the hand movement so that you do not see all of the movement.

You try to alter the subjective time value of a medical or

dental experience. But it is so very, very nice to experience very pleasant things, and so in medical and dental hypnosis you want the patient to lengthen, to increase, the time values of those things that are pleasant.

You tell the child, "I put the needle through the skin so fast that you can scarcely see it, and now you can take such a nice, long, slow breath in between the stitches."

And so you suggest a long, long period between stitches. there is no penetration of the skin at the breathing intervals—"nice, long, deep breaths"—and so by your method of altering that suggestion you increase the pleasant, pleasurable, subjective time values of whatever the medical procedure is. When the dentist says, "Now lean *slowly* forward and empty your mouth so carefully," the patient does it. His attention is on that pleasant intermission of emptying his mouth. Even a slight touch on the shoulder can move the patient's body forward at an increased rate of speed, because he is concentrating on *the subjective time values.*

I taught that cancer patient the shortness of time, subjective time, in experiencing his pain. I also taught him a prolongation of time for that period when he was freed from pain. But I didn't tell him that he was *free from pain:*

"It seems a long time that you're feeling so comfortable."

I didn't mention pain, why should I? I wanted him to have amnesia:

"It seems so long that you have been resting comfortably."

I wanted him to have amnesia:

"It seems so long that your leg has been resting on that pillow, comfortably. Isn't it surprisingly long to you, that duration of comfort?"

Build up time values in your patients that meet their particular situations.

Inducing Hypnosis

The Fractional Approach to Facilitating Hypnotic Induction: Enlisting "Just a Little" Patient Participation; Building up Trance "One-Thousandth of an Inch"

Recall the obstetric patient who said that the duration for her muscle contraction was such a nice, long, comfortable experience; and that every time it came to such a quick ending she was always surprised. And it did surprise her each time. First she had prolongation of subjective time to experience the contraction of the muscle. And then as the contractions got stronger and stronger, time shortened for her. And so she gave all of her subjective appreciation to the milder aspects of the labor contraction, and very little subjective time value to the stronger part of the muscle contraction.

Now having taught a patient something about subjective time values and amnesia for pain, then I can take up with him this matter of anesthesia and analgesia. Too often in medical and dental hypnosis you endeavor to drive ahead and to accomplish too much.

Take the highly resistant patient who says, "I'm sorry, a lot of doctors have tried to put me into a trance and failed, and I don't think you can put me in a trance either." And you could agree with the patient that you cannot, but you wonder if he learned one-thousandth of one percent of how to go into a trance; or was it two-thousandths of one percent of a trance? Now patients are willing to admit that they have learned one percent of how to go into a trance. It's such a little thing, a minimal amount. What do you want of your patients? You want a willingness to accept and to respond *just a little*.

Folklore is full of examples of that sort. You all know the story of the camel and the Arab in the sandstorm.

"Please, master," said the camel, "my nostrils are very tender. May I put them inside the tent?... Please, master, my eyes are very tender, may I put them inside the tent?... Please, master, my ears, my neck, my shoulders, are very tender..."

It wasn't long before the Arab was outside of the tent, the camel was inside the tent, and now the *Arab* was saying, "Please, camel, my nose is very tender... may I put it inside the tent?"!

You give a fraction of an inch, a thousandth of an inch, then you move on to two-thousandths of an inch, to four- and to eight-thousandths. Just make sure that you build it up in the patient.

The patient states, "Well, undoubtedly I could develop a *light* trance." And your statement should be, "Well, if it's really necessary, let's make it a rather light trance." And then his reaction will be to go all the way into a full trance. Always be aware of human nature, of the willingness of your patient to cooperate.

Why should you force your patient? Why not let the patient have the opportunity of participating in this matter of the use of hypnosis. You see, that is one of the things that is too often overlooked in medical and dental hypnosis: the tremendous importance of getting your patient to participate. Who are you that you should take charge of the situation? The important thing is to have the patient join in so that you are accomplishing a common goal, achieving a common purpose, a purpose that belongs to both of you—you, as the professional, and the patient as the patient. You need his cooperation, and therefore you never try to force or push unless he asks you to—unless he really demands it of you—and then you obediently do as he tells you thereby setting an example.

Inducing Hypnosis

An Authoritative-Participation Approach to Trance Induction

I can think of a doctor's daughter who came in and told me: "Now, listen, my father is a doctor. He's very autocratic, very dictatorial. All of my life I've been used to him giving orders. I've watched you use hypnosis, and you tend to do it softly and gently, and I don't go for that. When you talk to me, talk to me as if you meant it, the way my father would!"

Therefore, having received my orders, I stood over her and said: "Go into a trance without any further loss of time!"

Well, *that's* what she asked me to do. I was very obedient. But she set the pattern, and she participated, and *I* took my orders. Having demonstrated my capacity to receive those orders, she was bound psychologically to demonstrate *her* capacity to do the same. I could follow orders, and so could she. In this way it became a participation on her part and on my part.

Too often the orientation tends to be, "Now this is what I'm going to do to you," rather than a matter of "What will we do together?". When the patient finally recognizes that he might go into a trance, you ask for a *light light* trance; then he has the opportunity of volunteering a *light* trance. Then you can be willing to settle for the light trance, even though he might like to go into a *medium* trance. And you raise that issue. You are ready to settle for the light trance, even though the patient is willing to go into a *light medium* trance, and the patient wonders why he shouldn't go into a *medium* trance. And again you have offered him an opportunity of cooperating and participating with you in the entire procedure.

Pain Control in Hypnosis

Utilizing a Fractional Approach to Reduce Pain; Setting Limits via the Negative to Discharge Doubt and Increase Motivation

When I asked the cancer patient to accept the idea of a diminution of his dull, throbbing, continuous pain by one-thousandth of one percent, he said that that ought to be easy—just one-thousandth of one percent of that dull, throbbing, continuous pain. And I pointed out to him that he probably would not be able to perceive the diminution of one-thousandth of one percent. He admitted it would be difficult, and then he said he would put it up to five-thousandths of one percent. Now he was the one who mentioned the five-thousandths of one percent. I wanted him to mention that increase, and I gave him every opportunity. He was telling me what diminution he would be able to recognize. And that patient was oriented in all of his desires to a diminution of his dull, aching pain. He had amnesia for his lancinating pain. And together, the two of us worked it out: one percent, up to ten percent, up to twenty percent. Then I raised the question, "Do you know that we can't go beyond eighty percent?" The issue became the difficulty of *surpassing the eighty percent* of his pain.

You see, you need to know what you want to achieve. I wanted to free that patient of all the pain possible. I started by accepting a minimum percent of decrease and then let it build up to five percent, to a more noticeable ten percent, and then I raised a strong difficulty: the impossibility of surpassing eighty percent removal of his pain. A totally different problem. Then I was going to deal with only twenty percent of the pain, and the question became, "Could I do anything at all about that twenty percent?"; eighty percent had already been accounted for.

Pain Control in Hypnosis

Utilizing Dreams and the Interrelationship of Psychological Processes to Facilitate a Hallucinatory Dissociation: Reviving and Altering Past Experiential Learnings for Anesthesia

That is the sort of fractional approach you try to make. Now, I am stressing all of this because I want you to appreciate that in the scientific development of hypnosis you need to examine every one of these problems; you need to analyze them and to understand what sort of an approach you are going to make. The cancer patient had this idea of anesthesia and analgesia, but then the issue came up that there are other psychological processes involved. Just as the toe bone is connected to the footbone, the anklebone is connected to the leg bone, and so on, so is amnesia connected to memory, and so is memory connected to feeling, and so is feeling connected to no feeling, and so is no feeling connected to pain, and so is pain connected to position sense, and so is position sense connected to your appreciation of how you are placed in reality. All of your psychological processes are interrelated against a general background of total influx of symptoms and total analysis of those stimuli that you are receiving.

So with this dying man I raised the question of whether or not he could feel the pain over there in that corner of the room. Inasmuch as he was in bed, I didn't think he could feel any pain out there in the livingroom. He gradually began to get my idea: *Now, of course, when I am in bed I certainly cannot feel pain in another room in another position.* Then I pointed out to him the importance of understanding that in his dreams at night he could be in bed, in a boat, in an airplane, in the woods; he could be swimming, he could be visiting friends, he could be any number of other places experiencing all sorts of subjective reactions. In his dreams he could use the type of memory, the type of thinking, that belongs to the unconscious. So he could dream that he was driving an automobile and he certainly would not feel a bed or a pillow or the head of the bed or the railing inside the bed, because in the dream he would be in an automobile, and he would be utilizing the visual, mental images of an automobile, drawing upon past experiential values to compose the images in the dream. *Past experiential values are as genuine as any reality can be.* And that is an important consideration that you need to keep in mind in conveying understandings and ideas to patients.

Just shortly before leaving Phoenix, I called upon a patient of mine and had her describe all of her feelings as she sat in the livingroom. Actually she was in bed. She gave me an extremely vivid account of all the feelings she had in a wheelchair in her livingroom. Now, do you suppose she could feel any of that continuous, dull, aching pain from the cancer in her hipbone, in her spine, while she was telling me exactly what it was like to sit in a wheelchair; exactly how the arms of the wheelchair felt; exactly where the back of the wheelchair rested against her spine; exactly the position of her eyes when viewing the television screen; and exactly how much she could see with her peripheral vision from the wheelchair? She could not, because she was too interested in the revival of those experiential learnings about sitting in a wheelchair. And, of course, she was literally dissociated from her pain as she described sitting in that wheelchair.

So in inducing an anesthesia for pain you want to induce it not only by amnesia, not only by anesthesia and analgesia, not only by alteration of subjective time values, but *by an alteration of subjective, sensory learning and experience.* This woman forgot about the pain in bed; it was as if she were out in the livingroom watching television, seeing the screen door that led to the street, looking at the flowers over on the end table, seeing me sitting there on the couch in her livingroom. She had a very, very complete, pleasurable dissociation.

Pain Control in Hypnosis

Progressive Suggestions for Dissociation: Systematic Utilization of Subjective Time Values, Implication, and Somatic Interrelationships

But, you see, in building up that dissociation in the first place, you have to start bit by bit:

"I wonder if you can tell me a small bit about how your arm feels when it rests on the arm of the wheelchair?"

I knew what I was driving at, and the patient wanted to cooperate with me even though she didn't know what I was driving at. The patient wanted to cooperate by telling me every bit she could remember about the sensations of her hand on the arm of that wheelchair. Then, of course, I could proceed to the matter of the right foot on the footrest. Now it's important to mention the right foot because that indirectly implies that later it will be the left foot: "This is what you do now in relationship to your right foot."

It is a matter of offering suggestions. You need to have an awareness of all the things you want to do, and you introduce them very carefully and very systematically. If I am going to produce dissociation in that woman, if I am going to produce dissociation in that man, both dying of cancer, I had better get hand sensations going, subjective values going; then I had better get the right foot, because it was the right hand that I started with; then I had better get the left foot by implication, and then I have got from one end of the patient to the other end of the patient. The man had cancer of the prostate, the woman had cancer of the uterus with metastasis of the hipbone, so I worked from this end to that end, converging in the middle. The patient didn't know it, but I knew it. It is a matter of your own willingness to view your patient rather completely and comprehensibly.

Priorities in Symptom Correction

Treating the Outer Manifestation Before the Underlying Cause; Indirect Approaches in the Treatment of Trichotillomania: Hypnosis and Reframing via Distraction, Questions, and Wonder: "Which Would Grow Faster?"

The question reads: "What is your method of dealing with trichotillomania?"

Trichotillomania is that compulsive pulling out of the hairs of the head. You see it most often in children, and in adult cases you're most likely to find it in certain hysterical types, in certain psychotic types. This trichotillomania may be of the scalp, it may be of the eyebrows, it may be of the eyelashes.

Trichotillomania in children usually develops as a protest reaction of some sort. And then the parents immediately try to interfere, so the child demonstrates that he does own that hair and that he can pull his own hair out. And the parents say, "But you can't!", and the child says, "But I can!"—and proceeds to prove it over and over and over again. The entire issue becomes a source of combat between the parents and the child. And if the parents decide to take their child to a child guidance clinic, the child knows that he's being taken there to have his privilege of pulling his own hair out with his own hands taken away from him. So he goes in for it all the more strongly!

The best approach to the child with this sort of problem involves a willingness on the part of the parents to encourage the child to do that hair-pulling as long as it is necessary, and as long as it takes you to find out what all the feelings are. Now, just how long is the child going to waste his valuable time, because he soon explores and exhausts his learnings in this matter of hair-pulling. If it happens to be the eyebrows and eyelashes which the child is pulling, then you have another problem because the child hates the disfiguration. But as for that bald spot back here, the child does not concern himself. Your approval of this trichotillomania of the scalp allows the child to explore it. And you tell him, "You undoubtedly will have to keep on doing it for a number of months." But what is the child doing in the first place? He's showing you that he can do it, because you might interfere. And you are telling him that he *has* to keep on doing it for another three or four months—perhaps longer. And you have told him that he will *have to* keep on pulling out his hair.

You see, as a psychiatrist *I do not think there is much to be gained from analyzing the underlying cause before you correct the symptomatic manifestation. You do not want to be searching for the underlying cause while the symptomatic manifestation goes on and aggravates the underlying cause.*

Another approach is to ignore the matter altogether and instead get the child interested in different types of haircuts. Is the little girl old enough to wear a ponytail, or is she old enough to wear a braid? Is she really old enough to wear French braids? And you debate those questions seriously and earnestly, and you ought to take them seriously in your own mind. Your debate is not to be a pretense, because, you see, here is a child who has not yet become oriented to hair. Therefore you can raise the questions honestly, legitimately, sincerely: Is the child old enough to wear French braids?... Is the child old enough to wear ordinary pigtails?... Is the child old enough to wear a ponytail?... Is the child old enough to wear bangs? These are sincere and honest questions, because the child has already demonstrated that she is not oriented to this matter of hair on the head. And you want the child to be oriented to the hair on the head. Then you can take up any deep, underlying problems.

>Eds: In these two paragraphs Erickson is clearly indicating how he believes the traditional analysis of underlying

causes before symptom change can be reversed by first reframing the symptomatic behavior into constructive goals—and *then* "you can take up any deep underlying problems."

But, as I said, when the child is pulling out the eyebrows or the eyelashes you have a different kind of problem. I would try to enable the child to make an utterly, completely, laborious task out of the habit. And how can you make a laborious task out of pulling the hairs out of the eyebrows?

"You know, you really ought to pull one here, and then exactly halfway pull out another, and then all the way and pull out another. And then you start over there, and there, and there, and there. And then you build up a rhythm, a pattern, an alteration. And really, you know, it should be done as a part of your growing up—for as long as you need to do it. And you ought to do it in the best possible way. Now this is my idea. But maybe you can figure out another way."

You enlist the child in figuring out some way of pulling out the hairs of the eyebrow. You do not deprive the child of the right to dispose of his own eyebrows, but you help the child to work out a satisfactory way. What happens? The child works out a way, and you approve, and the child basks in your approval.*
But once a systematic, orderly way of doing it is worked out, and the child commits himself to it, it then becomes a tedious task. It's something that he wants to fudge on. He'll skip it today, and then he'll forget about it tomorrow, and why did you bring it up in the first place? He's busy doing something else. In other words, the child begins to want to shed that laborious task.

The same procedure works in the case of eyelashes. I can think of one little girl who had completely bare eyelids. Not a single eyelash. And I told her that a lot of people thought her eyelids looked homely—but *I* thought that they looked interesting. And the girl was pleased, and she believed me. But I *did* think that her eyelids looked interesting, because I was viewing it from the child's point of view.

**Editors' Note:* Notice that Erickson is indirectly giving the child an experience of relating positively and cooperatively to an adult.

Then I raised the question of would her eyelids look even more interesting if she had one eyelash here and one over here. And the next question was, what about one in the middle—three eyelashes? How long would they be, and would the middle one grow faster than the outside ones? That became another interesting problem about which I was enthusiastic. Did the eyelashes on the left eyelid grow faster than those on the right? Well, how do you answer that question except by letting them grow? And I was interested in the growth. But the girl knew that I was interested in her ideas, and with my aid she built up a number of interesting ideas.

The question that usually comes up is, *when did I hypnotize her? I hypnotized her when I distracted her attention, when I fixated her attention, and when we dealt with the question of the growth of the eyelashes on her eyelids.* She wasn't thinking about the tricycle in the backyard, about the little doll in the bedroom, about the play dishes, about mother's scolding or father's disgust, or anything. *She was just tremendously interested and absorbed in this question* of her eyelashes and their patterns of growth—which would grow faster?

Indirect Approaches in the Treatment of Scalp Ulcers

Utilizing the Patient's Viewpoint and Need for Accomplishment to Reframe the Problem via Paradoxical Questions: "Which Hand Gets Better Results?"

The next question is: "What do you do with adults who scratch their heads until they ulcerate the scalp, and then continue to keep that ulcer there by constantly picking at it?"

I think the answer is just what I pointed out for trichotillomania. Most of those problems are similar. You need to view them from the patient's point of view. Never mind what you as a medical person think about ulcers—you keep your private opinions to yourself. You can understand your own opinions adequately, whereas your patient cannot. But you do need to understand what the patient thinks, and what the patient feels, and how the patient wants that particular problem. Then the question is one of how to aid the patient in having all the satisfaction of an ulcer on his scalp.

What legitimate satisfaction do you get from an ulcer on the scalp? You can get a tremendous satisfaction from knowing that you had an ulcer on your scalp and that it got well, bit by bit. There is a sense of accomplishment in that. Consider the tremendous sense of accomplishment in that little girl as she measured the comparative growth of the eyelashes I had scattered on her right and left eyes. Then there was that 26-year-old man with a Masters Degree who really enjoyed watching his fingernails grow back. It is the same sort of approach. You try to set up a situation that allows the actual orientation of the patient to change for his benefit. And you do not do it by a massive enforcement of common sense, because if patients had all the common sense they needed, you would have to look elsewhere for your office rent! [Laughter]

I would want the child who picks at scalp ulcers to tell me if he got better results digging at his ulcers with his right hand or his left hand... decisions, decisions, decisions! Who wants to make all those decisions? The child doesn't know the answer. Does he get better results picking at his ulcers in the morning? ... mid-morning?... noon?... mid-afternoon?... late afternoon?... early evening?... going to bed? I know the history of the fact that he does dig at those ulcers, *but I've raised these other questions which alter the entire picture.*

If the child picks at his scalp just before he goes to sleep, I would want to have that knowledge before I raised any questions. I would want to know if he had tried to find out if it was more satisfactory just after breakfast. And it would be a sincere inquiry, and I would want him to make a sincere investigation. You see, *you use hypnosis not as a curative agent, but as a means of getting your patient to alter his behavior in a beneficial way. You do not deprive him of his behavior, but you aid him in changing it and varying it.*

Eds: This is another clear expression of how Erickson began to develop and teach the concept of reframing ("altering the entire picture"), which is becoming popular in psychotherapy only now, about a generation later.[4]

Indirect and Direct Approaches to Stop Smoking

Altering Orientations via "Not Knowing" and "Investigating":
Erickson's Painless Habit Cessation with the Help of the
Unconscious

Now here is a question full of barbs: "What methods were used by the panel members for giving up smoking?"

It should interest you to know that Dr. Secter hasn't given up smoking. He just doesn't know when he's going to smoke the next cigarette. It will probably be years and years from now, but he hasn't given up—he just *doesn't know* when he's going to smoke again!

Aston altered his smoking behavior by getting interested in how he would feel, what would happen inside him, if he swore off completely. He wanted to know how one would alter the habit. So he swore off smoking completely, and analyzed that experience, then he started in again, then he quit again, and so he was investigating this matter of alteration. And now he smokes one or two cigarettes on the way to the office and on the way home from the office, and that is a sufficiency for him.

As for me, I vowed that if a second AMA report came out even hinting that it might be advisable to quit smoking, I would quit. Inasmuch as I was the only smoker in the family, it was then very easy to do so. I just stopped one night after reading the second AMA report. The orientation I had was that once I had stopped, never again would I smoke another cigarette. That orientation saved me from all the peculiar, dry-mouthed hunger for cigarettes. My own unconscious, out of sympathy for me, repressed it! And I was very much surprised to find out that I didn't have a hunger for cigarettes.

I don't know how or why Seymour quit smoking, but I think he just got jealous of the halos the rest of us were wearing! [Laughter]

> Eds: This was a fascinating historical turning point for the entire staff and teaching faculty of the American Society of Clinical Hypnosis (ASCH). Most of the Society members were smokers. With the increasing medical knowledge of the harmful effects of smoking, they were all mutually challenged to use their own hypnotherapeutic methods to help themselves—indeed, "Physician, heal thyself." If they could not stop smoking, after all, how could they convincingly help their patients?
>
> The most interesting aspect of this *rite de passage*, however, was that it confirmed a fundamental shift in attitude away from the older, authoritarian view of hypnosis and toward Erickson's newer, permissive-utilization approach. For if all the faculty and staff of ASCH were generally of equal status and prestige, how could they impose their authoritative will and suggestions on one another to stop smoking? Authoritative suggestions can only work when there is a hierarchy of command; it is simply not effective in a democracy where all are equal.
>
> Instead, the faculty members could be interested in how their own unconscious minds would facilitate individual approaches to stopping smoking. Each faculty member could be interested in each other member's approach. This interest, together with the question of how each would do it—what particular shifts in mental orientation would be created—tended to *focus attention and suspend or depotentiate usual conscious attitudes. Inner searches could then be initiated, leading to everyone finding their own unique ways to stop smoking*. Thus it could be speculated that the initial conditions of the microdynamics of trance and suggestion[5] were operative within the entire group, facilitating the stopping of smoking via a form of creative group hypnosis.

One wonders if this could be a model of how group change can take place in a democratic setting: each group member facilitates the process by *questioning and wondering how his or her own unconscious will respond to the needs of the situation for change*, rather than attempting to impose one person's will over another for change. It appears that some religiously oriented groups (i.e., the Quakers in the West, and various Zen and meditatively oriented groups of the East) have hit upon this same approach from very different premises.

Note how very different this creative-receptive approach is from other current "democratic" styles of so-called debate, legalistic authoritative judgment, and power politics. In actual practice groups with democratic ideals fall into a wide range of effectiveness. At their best they have a receptive-creative relation to change and the new that is continually evolving by itself in a natural manner. At their worst they fall prey to mutually manipulative relationships wherein each individual or faction tries to impose its own limited world view on the other. It appears at this point in history that the proper focus of study for mankind is to learn to recognize and facilitate the conditions of the more desirable of these polar opposites in democratic institutions. In this area there is much fertile soil for the creative extension of Ericksonian psychotherapeutic and hypnotherapeutic approaches to these larger socio-cultural contexts.

Pain Control in Hypnosis

Indirect Hypnotic Techniques for Cancer Pain: Contingent Suggestions Tying Accomplishment to Continued Participation

Now the next question concerns the cancer patient: "What was the induction technique?" With cancer patients suffering a great deal of pain you need to use different techniques, because when they are in a lot of pain you need some kind of technique that can arrest their attention.

An 80-year-old man was dying of cancer. The pain could not be controlled with Demerol, morphine, or any other narcotic. He voluntarily discontinued the drugs for a day so that I could come over that evening and work with him. Since he was a professional man and knew a little about hypnosis (but had no personal experience with it), my statement to him was that it must have tired him immensely to experience all of that pain all day long, waiting and waiting for me to come over in the evening. It must have fatigued him horribly, and perhaps the best thing for him to do would be to take 20 minutes to a half hour of physiological sleep, and I would wait out in the other room and rest up myself.

That was my approach to him. Do you see the suggestion I was giving him?: that waiting and waiting all day, suffering so much pain, had tired him physiologically, and that *he had better take 20 minutes, a half hour, of physiological sleep.* I justified the rest on the basis of the day's experience, which was a legitimate basis for fatigue, a legitimate basis for taking 20 minutes, 30 minutes, of sleep. But, of course, as soon as he fell into physiological sleep, he did so in response to my request, and he therefore made a major response to my request. And when I gave him that suggestion, I also told him that after that 20 to 30 minutes of physiological sleep, he could awaken feeling perfectly rested as a result of that little catnap—a second hypnotic suggestion. He awoke about 20 to 25 minutes later, stating that he felt very much rested. Then I proceeded with my explanations of subjective values, anesthesias, and so on.

I also suggested that he develop *just a light trance* at first—not a deep trance, but *just a very light trance*—and we would take up the deeper trances later. So if he developed a very, very light trance, that meant he was committing himself to developing a deeper trance. You see, what I wanted him to do was *participate in a fashion that made further participation contingent upon his accomplishments, such that the more he accomplished the more he was committed to doing.*

Pain Control in Hypnosis

Vicarious Hypnosis to Overcome Resistance: Utilizing Distraction and Wishing Through the Agency of a Third Person: "Your Mother Ought to Be Free of Pain"

Another person I worked with, a gradeschool graduate, was very fearful of hypnosis. My approach to her was rather simple. I turned to her 19-year-old daughter and said, "Your mother really ought to be free of pain." The daughter couldn't possibly dispute me on that, but she was not quite certain of how she felt about hypnosis. But there was this one point on which we did agree: "Your mother really ought to be free of pain. And I wonder how much you are willing to teach your mother through your own, normal, healthy behavior." And so I stressed the daughter's normal and healthy behavior. And she expressed full willingness. Then I asked the girl if her father would be willing to assist me in teaching her mother how to be free of pain. And, of course, the girl said that her father would be willing, and indeed he was most willing. Then I wanted to know if the other sister would participate. And that meant I had a father and two sisters all willing to teach the woman to be free of pain.

I pointed out to the 19-year-old daughter that the best way to begin would be for her to discover that she could forget her hand. I patted her hand and told her that she could forget to feel the patting while she looked at her mother and wished that her mother would be free of pain. And, you know, she did wish intensely that her mother would be free of pain, and while she was wishing so intensely, how much attention was she paying to what I was doing to her hand? Her attention was completely distracted from her hand and redirected to a very intense, emotional issue.

Having set up that response, it was a relatively easy matter to put the girl in a trance—because I already had my anesthesia with her hand. So I put her in a trance, and the mother watched her daughter, and I saw to it that the mother had a very good appreciation of her daughter's trance behavior. I had the daughter demonstrate everything that I wanted the mother to learn, and the mother forgot about her pain in the interest with which she watched her daughter.

Hypnosis as the Communication of Needed Ideas

Unconscious Implication as a Therapeutic Bind: The Value of Family Participation for Teaching Purposes

Now, this woman I saw just before I came here had her master's degree. She was an exceedingly intelligent woman, with strong resistances to hypnosis. Her daughter was going to college, and it was a rather simple matter to enlist the daughter's interest.

The daughter said to me, "You can hypnotize Mother, but you can't hypnotize me." My reply was, "I'd like to have you tell that to your mother."

How many of you recognize what I said?: "I'd like to have you tell that to your mother." It's another way of saying, "Tell it to somebody else—*I* don't believe you." I asked her to tell it to her mother because I was rejecting her statement. So the girl told her mother, "He can hypnotize you, but I don't think that I can be hypnotized." She was in a bind right then and there, and she never even recognized what I did. The girl very promptly went into a nice trance, and then I used her to demonstrate for her mother.

> Eds: What is the actual bind in this case? The editors speculate as follows. When Erickson said, "I'd like to have you tell that to your mother," he was indirectly implying: "I don't believe you; I *can* hypnotize you." Thus the unconscious implication (and we know that unconscious implication is a most powerful method of suggestion) *"I can hypnotize you"* became associated with *"Tell that to your mother."* When the girl actually did tell that to her mother on a conscious level, she automatically and unconsciously

evoked within herself the consequent associated implication, *"I can hypnotize you."* She therefore "very promptly went into a nice trance," and served adequately as a demonstration subject for her mother. This is a brilliant example of how Erickson could evoke effective response-abilities in patients in a manner that was surprising and often contrary to their ego consciousness.

What is important is your willingness to use the other members of the family for teaching purposes—by visual instruction, auditory instruction, and to shut off resistances. You see, *hypnosis is always a matter of communicating ideas that your patients need. You must have a willingness to study each patient and his needs so that you can communicate the ideas that he needs to further his own purposes, and actually to achieve a corrected goal.*

Factors Disrupting Obstetrical and Dental Anesthesia

Subject's Needs Subserviated to Operator's; Erickson's Opposition to Stage Hypnosis; Covering All Possibilities of Response

[Now another panel member reads a question: "I had established a profound obstetrical anesthesia in my patient when, for no reason known to me, the anesthesia abruptly disappeared. Reinduction was unsuccessful. My question is, why did it disappear, and what could I have done about it?"

[Panel member answers the question by suggesting that the patient needed to recognize that the burden of a successful hypnotic anesthesia rested with her—was her project, so to speak. He also considers the possibility that the patient's resistance was triggered inadvertently in some minor way, resulting in the disruption of the anesthesia. He cites a case previously reported in the literature in which a hypnotist had achieved an excellent obstetrical anesthesia with a woman about to give birth. He then decided to make a display of the woman, as there were quite a number of hospital staff observing his work. He made the woman walk from the labor room to the delivery room, but while she was doing so, she began to scream "as if she were being killed." In other words, she forcefully rebelled once she realized that the hypnotist was using her for his own purposes. The panel member then cites one of his own cases involving a much less obvious action on the part of an obstetrician. Through a minor misunderstanding, the obstetrician made his patient feel uncomfortable, which then triggered her resistant tendencies. Now Erickson responds.]

I agree with Dr. Pattie. When you are working hypnotically with a patient, your orientation should center around the patient and the patient's needs. Whenever you try to maximize your own ego through a patient you start losing ground. *That is why we are so much opposed to the teaching of stage hypnosis techniques, because stage hypnotists are oriented about themselves as operators, not about their subjects.* In medical and dental hypnosis, you need to orient everything about the patient. It is the patient who is the important person.

Now there is one other technical point on this matter of losing an obstetrical anesthesia. Very often the answer can be found in the development of unexpected discoveries on the part of the patient. When a woman is having a baby, she has an understanding of the birth canal as an internal structure. Her doctor also may have described it to her as an internal structure, and therefore she expects all sensations, all reactions, to be internal in nature. So when the baby's head hits the perineum, the woman suddenly experiences external body sensations. But according to all of her previous understandings, birth is an internal process. So it seems to her that everything is going wrong, because there are these external sensations suddenly coming into play.

The dentist who develops an awfully nice anesthesia in the jaw of his patient overlooks the fact that he may touch the temporal area, which has nothing to do with the jaw so far as the patient is concerned. Or the dentist might accidentally brush his sleeve against the patient's ear. And, you know, the patient has been told that he's not supposed to feel anything while the dentist is working on him. Well, that's an inaccurate definition of things, because maybe he will feel things while the dentist is working on him. Maybe he will feel the dentist's sleeve against his ear, so the wise dentist defines the situation as one in which the patient isn't going to feel anything in his mouth—and then he covers for those unexpected stimuli so that they do not interfere.

My statement to patients is this: "A number of things may develop, some of which I have not mentioned. I hope you will notice and appreciate them, and then fit them into the goal that you wish to achieve. And I'd like to have you interested in the way these unexpected things can fit into the goal you wish to achieve."

With that type of appraoch, the dental patient can feel the dentist's sleeve against his ear and fit the sensation into the goal the dentist is working on. And it's all right for the dentist inadvertently to stimulate the patient's ear with his sleeve or his arm, or whatever it happens to be. What is important is the nature of your suggestions, your comprehensiveness in wording them, and the freedom which you give your patient in allowing him to understand the total situation.

The Interrelationship of Psychosomatic and Hypnotic Phenomena

Stimulating One Sensory Modality (Or Hypnotic Phenomenon) by Evoking Another: Interconnection of All Experiential Learnings

The next question is: "In the dissociation technique, how do you handle a patient who fails to develop past sensory experience, and how do you prolong the dissociated state?"

Regarding this matter of developing past experiential learnings, I published a paper on the interrelationships of psychosomatic phenomena in 1943.[6] The point of the paper was that if you want a patient to develop an anesthesia, sometimes you first have to give him an amnesia. I remember one experimental subject who had to forget a certain street address before he was able to develop an anesthesia. I can remember another subject who just couldn't hallucinate anything visually. So I wondered if she liked music. She did like music. And, "Would it be all right to listen to the music of the orchestra over there?" As the subject listened to the orchestra over there, I wondered what she thought about the appearance of the drummer. And she told me what she thought about the drummer, and so forth and so on.

You see, sometimes you will have to approach a visual hallucination through an auditory hallucination. In other words, the ear is connected to the eye, and vice versa. *All our experiential learnings are interconnected—they are not separate, discrete learnings.* You ought to have a willingness to find out if the patient can develop visual hallucinations by finding out if the patient can develop auditory hallucinations. Suppose that subject I just mentioned had failed to develop both visual and auditory hallucinations. I still could have asked her to feel that weight on her hand. And if she could hallucinate the weight on her hand, then I would ask her how big the weight was. That would bring into play either the matter of ten inches square or ten pounds—a visual value of size, or a kinesthetic value of weight. I find out a lot about my patients in that manner of relating one type of phenomenon to another.

Prolonging the Dissociated State

Interspersing Permission to Disrupt It When Needed

Regarding the second part of that question, "How do you prolong the dissociated state?" I kept the man who was dying of cancer dissociated a good deal of the time. How long? Well, whenever I went away on a trip I would dissociate him completely from his hips (that was where he had the most pain), but I also gave him permission to get his hips back any time he needed them back. Thus the man was able to use his hips when he absolutely needed to, but he was also glad to relinquish them.

Another example is the woman I mentioned earlier. I dissociated her legs to the other bed on the other side of the room. She didn't need her legs until she got into her wheelchair briefly in the afternoons. Then she would get her legs back from the other bed and put them in the wheelchair. And when she got the wheelchair out into the other room, she would lose the sensation of her legs being in the wheelchair—because they would be back on the other bed again! You see, you can suggest all these things, but you also suggest that the patients can alter the situation any time, for as long as they need to do so. That way, you meet their needs.

Reframing the Presenting Problem in Learning Disabilities

Evoking Motivation and Personal Interests: Utilizing the Child's Control Over the Parent

Another question here concerns reading problems. I can think of the young boy who was brought in to see me. He belonged in the fifth grade, but he couldn't even read the first-grade reader. His parents had hired a tutor every summer, after he had been promoted to the next grade by the goodheartedness of the teacher.

The boy came into my office very resentfully. As soon as I got rid of his parents I said, "You know, I'm puzzled about something. Your parents think that I should treat *you,* but I think that I should treat *them,* because they have mismanaged this whole thing."*

The boy looked at me, wondering if I meant what I said. I continued. "Your parents want me to teach you to read, and you know darn well that you can't. You've had plenty of experience, you've had all the tutors. Shall we waste our time on that, or shall we have a good time? Your parents are paying me for my

---

Editors' Note: Here MHE reframes the presenting problem.

time, and you don't care about that. Shall we have a good time?"

He looked at me a bit questionably, and I added, "It will be an honest, good time."

"Okay," he said.

"Where would you like to go on vacation?" I asked. "You know, unfortunately I left my glasses out in the other room. And I wanted to study the maps and look up places with you."

We were *looking* at a map—we weren't *reading* a map. That is an important distinction. The boy and I examined this map and that map. Whereabouts in the Western United States should he go on his vacation? Now, let's see... Where is Yellowstone Park?... Where is Yosemite Park?... Where is Olympic Park? ... What city is it near?... Which highway goes from Yellowstone Park down to Grand Canyon? And so on. We never did *read* the maps; we *examined* the maps.* At each session we examined all kinds of maps, planning that vacation, and I always misplaced my glasses just before we began. But I wasn't fooling that boy. He knew unconsciously that I was giving him a face-saving method of learning how to read.

That September when school opened I told the boy's parents not to annoy him any further. They were to take him to school, and he would deal with the teacher himself. So when the teacher said, "Well, Tommy, what are we going to do with you?", Tommy answered, "The first thing you're going to do is give me a first-grade reader; then give me a second-grade reader, a third-grade reader, a fourth-grade reader, a fifth-grade reader." The teacher very obediently did as she was asked, and Tommy proceeded to read the first-, second-, third-, fourth-, and fifth-grade readers. Then he hauled out of his pocket a newspaper clipping about his father and their vacation trip, and he read it to the teacher. That was Tommy's solution.

You see, you enlist the aid of the child; you meet the child instead of trying to force him to recognize that c-a-t spells *cat*, and that d-o-g spells *dog*. The child already knows that, but he

---

*Editors' Note: Here Erickson reframes the problem area of *reading* into a fun activity of *looking* and *examining*.

has a mental block. Your task is to make it easier for the child to circumvent his own blocks. When Tommy and I began examining those maps, we were just having a good time. We were planning a vacation trip which I had promised his father would take him on, but *we* were mapping out where they would go. *That was a positive way of utilizing the boy's control over his parents.* Now they were planning a vacation, whereas before they were arranging for futile tutoring sessions.

A Brief Approach to Obesity

Suggestions Establishing the Preferability of "Small Portions"

It's almost noon and time for a break. I'll answer one more question quickly. The question is, "What do you tell the obese patient?"

I'll give you an example. I hope that everyone of you enjoys your lunch today. And I'd like to have you enjoy it thoroughly and well. You know, it's just as easy to enjoy a small portion as it is a large portion. In fact, those of you who eat a small portion will enjoy a small portion much more than you would a large portion. And you really will, because you won't even have to feel guilty about that small portion. You'll be perfectly delighted with it. And so, good appetite! [Laughter]

Erickson's Early Experiments in Anesthesiology

Using the Trance State to Recover Memories of Operating Room Events: Remarks of a Nasty Surgeon: Erickson's Conscious Experience of Anesthesia

[Tape resumes with Erickson in the middle of a topic. By way of introducing his topic of the degree to which the anesthetized person can respond, Erickson uses the analogy of the opossum, a creature known for its ability to appear dead when threatened.

Yet obviously the opossum is perceiving everything around him. Erickson then uses the example of the newborn human infant.]

In the human infant, newly born, vision is a rather complex matter. It's awfully difficult for it to see, and I doubt if the newborn infant really sees. I doubt if the newborn infant really feels, in a recognizing fashion—because it has no background of understandings. But there is one thing that the newborn infant can do: if you make a loud sound, it will respond. And very, very early in infancy, if you drop a baby the loss of weight in the process of falling can stimulate it. Loud noises and a sense of falling will elicit startle responses in the very young infant.

> Eds: Recent research in infant development presents a somewhat different view of the newborn's sensory and affective capabilities. While it is true that hearing is more developed than vision at birth, the newborn's range of responses is now known to be far more complex than was recognized at the time of this presentation.

Therefore, one wonders how patients under anesthesia respond: how much stimuli do they receive? They're not likely to see too much; they're not likely to feel too much, or you wouldn't be using an anesthetic and conducting an operation.

When I was in medical school I became interested in this question of what hypnosis can do, and how you can use it to uncover memories and discover things. In those days, I talked extensively with Ralph Waters, whom I regard as the father of American anesthesiology; I talked with William Lorenz, Professor of Psychiatry at the University of Wisconsin; and I talked with Levenhard, Professor of Pharmacology. These men were tremendously interested in research on human behavior. And they tolerated me, actually acting as protectors of my interest in hypnosis in those medical school days.* And we discussed a great number of things.

*Editors' Note: Presumably this comment refers to the fact that Erickson's superiors officially forbade him to practice hypnosis while he was in medical school.

Then when I became an intern I was interested in what an anesthetized patient really knows about what is going on during the operation. Do sound waves travel along a specific nerve to a specific center of the brain, if there is such a mechanism for the perception of sound? I soon found out one thing: by inducing trances in patients post-operatively, some of them were able to provide lots of information about what went on during their operations.

The details of what they selected to recall were remarkable. There was one surgeon who had a nasty operating-room manner. In the ward he was a charming gentleman, but in the operating room—well, I wanted to slaughter him many a time! (I often gave the anesthesia for him. We used ether, and the patients were under a deep anesthesia.) While he was operating on a patient, this particular surgeon would use the most uncomplimentary terms: he would describe the abdomen as a mountain of fat, for instance, or make insulting remarks about the body of a young girl—things of that sort. The remarkable thing was that patients who had this experience with the undesirable surgeon would tell me a good deal about what had happened in the operating room when they were later in the trance state. And they would remember those uncomplimentary remarks. But the patients who had had a surgeon who was reassuring throughout the operation did not recall his nice remarks. That gave me the feeling that a great deal is perceived and remembered, even in a deeply anesthetized state.

Since my internship days, I've run across similar instances time after time. I kept careful records of those cases I studied while an intern. I was very careful about watching the patient post-operatively so that nothing was said about the operating room events. And I knew what the surgeon had said in the operating room (because I had been there), so I could match it against the actual words that the patient in the deep trance would tell me had been said in the operating room.

There's one other comment that I want to make on this issue of anesthesiology. At some point during my work on the research service at Worcester State Hospital in the 1930's, I had to have an abscessed tooth opened, drained, and extracted. Dr. F, who was in charge of medical services and a good friend of mine, offered to act as the anesthesiologist. Arrangements were made with the dentist, Dr. B, who was also a good friend of mine. And, of course, since I was going to go under an anesthetic, we all agreed to find out what I would remember. Dr. B promised to keep a very, very careful record throughout the entire procedure.

Dr. B went about keeping his record and feeding me the ether-drop method of anesthesia, when finally he remarked: "He must be a secret faker. I've fed him two cans of ether already, but now I'm sure he's completely out." My remark was, "The hell you say!" [Much laughter] Then Dr. B said, "Well, I'll give you another can." The next record he made on the chart was of his statement: "That's three cans of ether—more than any human being can take at this altitude. *Now* he's out!" [Laughter]

After I'd come out of the recovery room, Dr. B asked me, "Well, what do you remember about your operation?"

"I kidded you, and I kidded the dentist," I replied.

"What exactly did you say?" Dr. B asked. And as he looked at his chart, I was able to tell him what he had written down while I was "completely out."

I think all of you ought to bear that in mind. You ought to recognize that the functioning of the human brain, the human mind, is something about which we know very, very little. We ought to have a tremendous interest in every experimental study and experimental inquiry being conducted. And I'm delighted with Dr. Cheek's paper.[7]

Indirect Approaches to Patient Reassurance

Implicative Requests Utilizing Promise and Contingency to Establish Inevitability of Recovery

Dr. Keat mentioned another issue in the matter of indirect reassurance. It's awfully nice, and awfully courteous, and very polite of you to tell a patient, "Of course you'll get well; most certainly you'll get well." What else could you be expected to say socially? It's only a social gesture. But if you really want to reassure the patient, you need to give him something more than a socially accepted verbal gesture of, "Of course you'll be all right." Why not make the patient promise to give you her recipe for son-of-a-gun stew just as soon as she gets home? (In case you don't know what son-of-a-gun stew is, you've really missed a treat!) [Laughter] *You ask patients to do something that is contingent upon their complete recovery and their return home.* In that way they think that you are selfishly asking them to give you a recipe, or that you are selfishly asking them to share their gladiola bulbs with you—something that is just for your benefit. *But it implies, of course, that they are going to get well,* they are going to go home, they are going to dig up some bulbs in their flower gardens, and they are going to share recipes with you. And so they have a sense of sharing their recovery with you.

[Erickson now discusses the topic of psychogenic infertility. This part of his 1958 presentation was edited into a paper entitled, "A Clinical Experimental Approach to Psychogenic Infertility," and published for the first time in Volume II of *Collected Papers* (pp. 196–202).]

PART III

NEW FRAMES OF REFERENCE FOR OLD*

Treating Obesity

A Therapeutic Double Bind to Overeat Sufficiently

Here is a question addressed to me: "Please describe the double bind and its usefulness in hypnosis. What qualities are necessary for its presentation?"

The quality you need in presenting the double bind is simplicity: you need to use a simple, straightforward presentation of the double bind. What is meant by the double bind? I can think of the 270-pound woman who came to me for the treatment of her obesity. She explained: "My husband is a doctor. I've been on plenty of diets, and he has sent me to all of his medical friends. I know more about dieting than the entire medical profession, yet every diet fails. Now my husband has sent me to you for hypnosis, but I don't think I'm going to lose any weight."

"We can use hypnosis," I replied, "but if I use hypnosis for the treatment of your obesity, I want it understood that I will use it *my* way. I am the doctor; you are just the patient. You ought to understand what that means as a doctor's wife. And since you worked in your husband's office, where you were just a receptionist and not a wife, you know how patients should be treated. A patient is a patient, and the doctor is the doctor."

---

*Meeting of The American Society of Clinical Hypnosis in Chicago, Illinois on October 8, 1959.

She agreed, but she also added: "I'm not sure I'll cooperate with you, because I always go off my diet and I always overeat!"

My statement was rather simple. I said: "All right. Your weight is 270 pounds (she was in a trance state). And I want it distinctly understood that I want you to do exactly as I tell you. Bearing in mind that you now weigh 270 pounds, *I want you to overeat throughout the week enough to support 260 pounds.*" A double bind: she was bound to lose and she was bound to overeat.

She returned in a week's time very much amused, laughing, and weighing in at 260 pounds. She said she had overeaten quite nobly! Then I told her that she was to overeat enough to support 255 pounds during the following week. In a little more than 40 days she had lost 40 pounds, and was still losing. That's one example of the double bind.

Treating Premature Ejaculation

A Therapeutic Double Bind Reversing the Problem: A Time-Limited Inability to Ejaculate

I can think of the patient with the problem of premature ejaculation. As I listened to this man's story—and it was a long, long sad story—I pointed out to him that *I didn't know which was the worse condition: premature ejaculation, or the impossibility of getting an ejaculation.* I admitted that he was in a sorry fix, because *sooner or later he would experience the development of the opposite condition.* Then I built up that idea in the trance state for him—the transformation of his premature ejaculation into the opposite condition of the inability to have an ejaculation—and attached a double bind to it. How? I explained to him that on his next occasion of intercourse following the interview, he would most likely experience an inability to have an ejaculation until at least 27 minutes had elapsed. Why 27 minutes? It makes one wonder, and I wanted my patient to wonder in his own mind why I picked out 27 minutes. I didn't want him to analyze the ideas I was presenting to him.

The result: on that particular night he had sex relations with his wife, wearing his wristwatch! [Laughter] And he couldn't possibly have that ejaculation until at least 27 minutes had elapsed, but at the end of 27 minutes he had the ejaculation. He reported the outcome to me the next day. I replied that time was an inconstant thing: it might take him 37 1/2 minutes to ejaculate the next time. I just wasn't sure. [Laughter]

But you see, I put him in a double bind in which he had to do something; he had to fight against himself in both directions. The obese woman had to overeat, and at the same time she had to lose. She had to cooperate with me, and yet she had to overeat—which is contrary to the idea of reducing. Over and over again *you present ideas so that the patient achieves the desired result no matter which way he goes:* "I suppose you could see those flowers on the left side of the table, and I'd rather you didn't see them on the right side of the table." Again the question becomes one of a double bind. Is the person going to see the flowers on the left side of the table, the right side of the table? You see, it isn't a question of *whether* he's going to see the flowers; it's a question of *where.* And he's caught in that double bind. He's bound to see the flowers, and he's bound to select the place where he sees them. Whenever you want to induce a condition in patients, you raise the possibilities.

Treating a Childhood Urinary Problem

Structuring a Therapeutic Metaphor out of Personal Goals: "Somebody's Got to Go to the Bathroom Sometime!"

What is the treatment for the child who just simply cannot endure the thought of using a school lavatory? I know one way I found to handle that problem. The child knew why he had been brought to see me, so that settled that issue. Both the child and I knew; therefore there was no need for any further discussion of the fact. Instead I began a casual conversation, and soon discovered that the boy was very interested in spaceships. I had some scratch paper and some pencils available, and I drew what I thought was an excellent design for a spaceship. We talked about my design, and the boy told me all about his ambitions to go on this sapceship. He agreed that I had drawn the correct design for such a spaceship. What had I done with my design? I had drawn in the shelves where you put the canned food, and then, of course, you have to figure out the number of days it would take to get to Mars, and here was just a one-room situation, and there were so many people aboard that spaceship. I let the boy take it from there. And in his own thinking he finally woke up to this fact: if it took that many days to get to Mars, and you ate all of that food, and there was just one room, and there were a lot of people in that room—well, somebody's got to go to the bathroom sometime! [Laughter] So if he was going to go on that spaceship someday, he might as well get acquainted with the idea of using public lavatories right now.

Why not do it that way instead of arguing and pleading and coaxing? Why not let the child do it in relationship to his own goals in life?

Treating an Adult Urinary Problem

Structuring a Physiological "Urgency" to Reverse Psychogenic Urinary Retention: A Case That Failed

Now back to the matter of cystitis and catheterization. A man brought his bride to me. They had been married a month when she developed a cystitis. They were referred to a physician who catheterized her. She had been catheterized daily for two weeks. Finally the physician got disgusted with the situation, and her husband brought her to see me.

She was a very nice hypnotic subject, and she listened to me very, very carefully. But I was afraid of the consequences, because I didn't quite feel that she was being fair and honest with me. So I dismissed her from the office and told her husband to take his wife home *directly*—and I repeated that he was to take her home *directly*.

The man started directly home with his wife, but on the way she said, "You know, I wonder if we could get a plant for Mother at Norman's Nursery. It isn't very far out of the way." And the husband responded, "Well, I'm supposed to take you directly home, but it's just two blocks out of the way, so it will be all right."

He took her to get the plant for Mother, which brought her directly in front of St. Joan's Hospital. She said, "I might as well go in and get catheterized now." That settled the therapy I had attempted!

What was the therapy? It was the same approach I published previously. How many of you have been at the theater and felt the need to go to the bathroom, but decided to wait until you got home? You drive all the way home and things are all right. Then you walk up to the front porch, you start fumbling for those keys, and you feel more and more urgency; you fumble the key into the keyhole, and in that last mad rush you dash to get to the bathroom in time! [Laughter] That was the situation I attempted to build up for this patient. I wanted her to get increasingly impatient to get home, and to feel threatened that she would wet her pants before she got there. But she outsmarted me with that resistance!

Now you can use that same sort of situation with the child who cannot use the lavatory at school. You build up an urgency situation where the question isn't, "Should I go to the lavatory?"; the question is, "Do I get wet pants, or what do I do?". And so the debate is on that question, not on the question, "Should I go to the lavatory?"

Brief Training in Autohypnotic Techniques

Relying Upon Unconscious Direction

The next question is, "Will you teach us to utilize autohypnosis on ourselves?" Yes, I can discuss it very quickly, very briefly.

Sit down in a chair, relax, close your eyes, and just be willing to let things happen. *You see, your unconscious mind is a lot more intelligent than you are. You aren't going to get very far if you try to direct it, because you would be directing it at the conscious level.*

So the best approach is to relax, close your eyes, and be willing to let things happen in terms of your own unconscious thinking, in terms of your own unconscious needs. You don't know consciously what your unconscious mind regards as important.

Training in Time Distortion

Utilizing Everyday Examples for Rapid Learning: Utilizing the "My-Friend-John" Technique for Self-Instruction

The next question is, "Please describe the use of time distortion and the kinds of verbalization used to induce it."

You do not have to use an awfully extensive verbalization for time distortion. Yesterday I gave just this amount of verbalization to subjects who had never before demonstrated time distortion:

"You are waiting for a bus on a cold, wet, rainy day. You're in an awful hurry to get downtown, and that bus is two minutes late. Your appointment downtown is important, and you've just got to be there on time. And waiting those two extra minutes for that bus seems like waiting all day. Then once it arrives, the bus seems to poke along all the way to town.

"Now it's a nice sunny day, and you're going downtown, and you're not in a hurry. A friend comes along and talks to you, and the bus is two minutes late the way it was the other time. But this time you're ready to swear that the bus is ten minutes ahead of schedule!"

With that amount of explanation I instructed my subjects: "Look at the movie screen back there and see a movie from beginning to end. I'm going to give you 10 seconds of waking time, but with the speed of thought you will see that movie slowly from beginning to end."

One of the subjects watched three-quarters of *The Ten Commandments,* and the other watched an hour-and-a-half show— I've forgotten the name of it. But those two subjects got no more explanation that what I described to you, and it was their first experience with time distortion.

You ought to use "my friend John" as a technique to train yourselves. There is John sitting in that empty chair over there, and you explain time distortion to him a few dozen times, and in a few dozen ways. You can use examples of waiting for a doctor to come in an emergency, waiting for the telephone to ring, etc. Don't always use the bus example. Try to explain time distortion to "my friend John," and you'll learn something about the proper verbalization.[1]

Developing Advanced Hypnotic Techniques

Observation, Examination, and Integration

I think our time is just about up. In closing, I would like to impress upon you just one point. In developing advanced hypnotic techniques you must emphasize the importance of examining your own awareness of ideas, getting the reactions of others to case histories, picking up an idea here and there, and integrating all of it into your own thinking and into your own practice. That is how you learn advanced hypnotic techniques: by carefully studying the ideas, the thoughts, the feelings of others, and picking up a little here and a little there.

Tomorrow will begin the second annual scientific assembly of The American Society of Clinical Hypnosis. I hope you will all attend.

Time Reorientation[2]

Therapeutic Manipulation of Subjective Time Experience: Utilizing Hindsight in the Present via Pseudo-orientation to a Future Perspective in the Resolution of Personal Problems

My paper is on pseudo-orientation in time, but I'm not going to read it to you. I prefer to offer you a few general statements about human behavior. You know, one of the most informative aspects of human behavior is this matter of hindsight. Hindsight is so awfully important, and you wonder why you didn't use this knowledge based on hindsight in the form of foresight. How often have you said to yourself, "If I had only known things would work out this way! I had all the data available to me beforehand, so why didn't I realize it would work out this way?" And in the practice of medicine and psychiatry, you need to speculate on how things are going to work out, and on how to use the available information.

The technique that I'm going to describe now is one which I have used for a good many years. The first step in the technique is this matter of the induction of a hypnotic trance—and usually a deep trance is employed. Then I ask the patient to reorient himself in time. Now that doesn't mean that I change calendar time or wordly time, but I ask the patient to alter his subjective understandings of time. We all have a general idea of what we will be doing next Christmas. We don't know exactly what we will be doing next Christmas, but we have certain general expectations. So I ask my patient to forget the immediate present and feel himself oriented instead to next Christmas or next year, so that he then can look back upon the "past." (Bear in mind that patients can be regressed in time or they can be progressed in time—both techniques can be employed toward this utilization of their capacities to think in various ways.) Then I ask the patient who has altered his time orientation to think comprehensively about stressful matters—about those things that worry him and make him fearful in his current life situation. And since he can look upon those things from his reoriented vantage point as having occurred in the past, he now can employ hindsight in their resolution! You see, hindsight is often no more than a focalization and utilization of the understandings that were available at the time the event occurred.

I also employ reorientation, pseudo-orientation, so that the patient, for example, can look forward to the eventual discovery that he's going to have a right-leg amputation. In actuality his leg has already been amputated, but I reverse the process so that he can look forward in time and focalize his personality forces [toward a complete and rapid adjustment].

What is the result of this sort of reorientation? I'm going to cite the case history of Edward and Jeanie to illustrate.

Edward and Jeanie had been married for five years, and they were very happily married so far as they themselves were concerned. They were childless—they said they didn't want children—but Edward's mother lived with them. Now Edward's mother was a very dominant woman, awfully dictatorial, awfully autocratic. And she really governed that household. Finally Jeanie said to Edward, "Either Mother goes or I go—there can't be two of us under this one roof!"

Edward came to me and asked what could be done about the situation. He loved his wife and he loved his mother, and he just simply couldn't kick his mother out of the only home she had. So in the trance state I asked Edward to discover that it wasn't the year of 1959—it was the year of 1965: "Can you tell me, Edward, exactly how things went along? How did it happen that you finally decided that your mother should leave your home and live by herself? Explain to me just how it came about and how she got along."

With all the fantasies and all the understandings Edward has acquired about his mother, he told me very simply: "You know, back in 1959 I didn't want to kick my mother out, but she made me. It was a most fortunate thing, because of all the things I knew about my mother, I knew that she was a very, very capable woman, able to adjust to the most difficult situation, always putting up a struggle with my father, always managing things in the best way possible. And you know the way these things happen... well, somehow my life with Jeanie also changed after my mother left our home. I can't exactly describe the changes, but our life changed for the better. Mother got along beautifully and her capacity for making friends helped a great deal."

After Edward came out of the trance having had that sort of discussion—and having developed an amnesia for trance events—I asked him to speculate with Jean and his mother about the situation, and to arrive at a nice conclusion. The result of their discussion was that Edward's mother came to the decision on her own. And she did make the good adjustment that Edward had expected, and Edward's life with Jeanie did change in ways he couldn't describe in the trance state: three children came along! And they had thought they were contented with being childless!

Over and over again I've asked patients to discuss how they would speculate upon the future if they viewed it as the past.

Time Reorientation

Reorientation to a Future Perspective in the Assessment of Birth Control Possibilities: Negative Results with Vasectomy as a Hypnotherapeutic Failure

Then there was the case of James and Joyce. They were 23 and 22 years old respectively. They had been married when Joyce was 16 and now had four children. They were having a tremendous row over whether she should have a self-protective hysterectomy or he a vasectomy.

I put them into a trance and projected them into the future, whereupon they both told me that they just simply couldn't tolerate the idea of the other being a "surgical cripple." That was their attitude, which they expressed to me most emphatically, when they were oriented to the future.

I awakened them from the trance state and asked them to speculate upon the possibilities available to them, and what they thought would happen. In discussing it they said that four children were enough at their ages, and that they had an adequate family. I let them discover, bit by bit, their feelings about this matter of being a "surgical cripple," and they laughed at me and rejected the idea. Finally they decided upon a vasectomy for the husband.

Two years after the vasectomy they came to me, very angry, and said: "You should have used more dominance in that conversation, and you should have prevented that vasectomy!" I told them that they were free citizens and that I couldn't, though I tried to, prevent it.

Time Reorientation for Personal Problem Solving

Reorientation to a Future Perspective to Assess Desirability of a Medical Hysterectomy: An Answer, and the Unexpected Activation of a New, Curative Viewpoint: Foresight Disguised as Hindsight

I can think of yet another excellent example of a woman who had had a history of eleven miscarriages. She had been advised to undergo a hysterectomy, so in the trance state I asked her what she really felt about that medical recommendation that she have a hysterectomy to prevent more miscarriages. She replied that she had obtained the best in medical advice. So then I asked her in the trance state how she thought she would feel looking back upon that hysterectomy, and I reoriented her several years into the future. Her statement was: "Each year that goes by with the knowledge that I have had a hysterectomy makes me feel more and more depressed. I just can't tolerate it. If I continue getting more depressed, as I have in the past few years, I will end up committing suicide." And she expressed all that quite convincingly.

After she had come out of the trance, I asked her to remember those things which she thought she ought to remember. She said: "You know, by going into a trance state I think I've discovered a new awareness of my body, and I'm going to look forward to this matter of the future in a different way. I don't think that I need to see you as a patient any longer. I've got a new attitude of hope. I'm not going to have a hysterectomy, but I am going to have an increasing amount of faith in myself."

There are now five children in that family. How they came about—except in the orthodox way—I don't know! [Much laughter] I can only speculate very, very vaguely upon the physiological changes that were mobilized to end that patient's tendency to miscarry. I've got about two dozen other similar cases that I could cite but I think the ones I've described are sufficient to give you the idea that you can *use hypnosis to focalize patients' thinking in such a way that they benefit from their own capacities for foresight—foresight disguised as hindsight!*

Establishing New Frames of Reference (Reframing)

Hypnosis as the Selection of Experiential Learnings and Functionings Already Present in the Individual

[You have all had the experience of being] so interested in a conversation that you reached your destination on the other side of the city without realizing that you had stopped for stoplights and that you had observed all the traffic laws. You just suddenly find yourself at your destination without even remembering how you got there. We all have unconscious learnings and unconscious functionings of that sort.

Do you remember the verse by Ogden Nash about the centipede who was asked which leg comes after which? When the centipede puzzled that question out, he fell into a ditch waving his legs, trying to figure out just which comes after which!

Did you ever try to tie somebody's bow tie? Even though you're an expert at tying one on yourself, now you just don't know your right hand from your left hand. You're an expert, yet you have to get behind the other person and pretend his neck is your neck in order to tie the bow tie. You see, *there are a tremendous number of learnings that we acquire at various levels of awareness, and whenever you do anything, you are aware of this part, aware of that part, and at varying levels.*

In the hypnotic trance you have the opportunity to search through your experiential learnings. Yet you also can do it in the ordinary waking state. Once when I was a boy at home on the farm, I was working in the barn one afternoon. I was hammering some nails. I suddenly realized that I needed something else, and that it was up on the back porch. I dropped the hammer and rushed up to the back porch. But on the way there, some other thoughts flittered through my mind, and I found myself up on the back porch wondering what it was I had come there to get. You've all had that sort of experience. Well, I looked all over the back porch and couldn't see anything I could possibly want in the barn. So I went back to the barn, picked up the hammer, hit a few licks on the head of the nail I had already driven in, and it came to me: I had gone to the back porch to get the hatchet. This time I kept my errand fully in mind as I went to the back porch, again! You see, when I returned to the hammering I was re-establishing the original setting and the original frame of reference.

Now in hypnosis you always try to induce your subjects to establish a different frame of reference so that they can function in that regard.* There are so many things, for example, that you know about your body functionings. If I asked you to alter your blood pressure, or to become warm or cold, you would look at me and wonder how to do that. Yet you could alter your blood pressure very, very quickly and very, very easily by having me utter just one single word in this room. And your blood pressure would change horribly. You might flush, you might turn pale with anger, because you've had plenty of experience in regard to vasomotor behavior. *In hypnosis you have the opportunity not of striving in a purposeful way, but in a way that allows you to select possible learnings. Just why that is, I don't know.*

> *Eds:* It comes as a relief that Erickson admits here that there is something about hypnosis that he does not know. Do we know anything more about this a generation later? We can confirm that hypnotic effects are indeed generated by "not striving in a purposeful way": that is, by not activating left-hemispheric logical, directed thinking. Hypnotic effects are probably mediated by the imaginative and symbolic processes of the right hemisphere. These imaginative and symbolic processes have more direct connections with brain-

---

*Eds: This is another clear expression of the concept of reframing which Erickson was developing during this time period.

mediated physiological processes via the limbic system and the hypothalamus. The new field of psychoneuroimmunology will probably serve as the new research base for future explorations in this area.[2]

Catalepsy in Psychosis and Hypnosis

A Motivational Differentiation Between Catatonic Schizophrenics and the Hypnotic Subjects: Purposive Versus Non-Purposive Behavior

There was another question raised in regard to catalepsy in the hypnotic patient and catalepsy in the catatonic schizophrenic. During my research at Worcester State Hospital Research Division on schizophrenia, I had the opportunity to question a good many catatonics once they had come out of their stupors. I also queried a good number of catatonics when I was later in Michigan. And I extensively questioned each one as to what the catalepsy was. Every catatonic who could give me an account always gave me an account which indicated that the catalepsy served some definite purpose. Now I don't know how to rationalize that. Albert, for example, did not move because if he moved the world would come to an end. Therefore he would remain in any posture you put him in: one leg with knee partly bent, head over to one side, one arm out in one direction, the other out in the other direction, and so forth. You could drop a light in front of him and mark out his shadow on the wall at eight o'clock in the morning. At four o'clock in the afternoon you again could mark out his shadow, and he still would be in that same, rigid, awkward, man-killing position. Yet as Albert later explained to me—he was a college man—he didn't dare move because he wished the world well! And every other catatonic I queried gave a similar, purposeful significance to the catatonia.

What about the normal subject I used yesterday in Galveston? I had a number of subjects on the platform with me to demonstrate hypnosis for the Texas Academy of General Practice. And here was this very nice nurse who sat very comfortably—I used her as the background for the other subjects—and she sat there very, very comfortably. Yet I had positioned her in a slightly awkward way, which I purposely had effected by clumsily rearranging her arms and her head a little bit. I let her sit there for about one hour in an absolutely perfect state of catalepsy. There were no movements; there was no behavior manifested whatsoever, except for that perfect catalepsy.

At the end of the hour, I asked her what she was doing. Her reply was that she was relaxing. Relaxation was her entire orientation; there was a withdrawal from all purposefulness in her activities so far as the maintenance of muscle behavior was concerned. She was relaxed, and later when I asked her about the catalepsy she said that it was the most restful experience she had ever felt in her life. As she was sitting in that cataleptic position, she wasn't aware of the awkwardness of it; she was only aware of *relaxation*. But the catatonic is *accomplishing* something with his catalepsy. He is either controlling the external environment or he is withdrawing from the external environment; but he is doing something purposeful in relation to the things external to him. The hypnotic subject merely rests comfortably within himself, in total peace, and without a need of utilizing his body in any particular way.

Varieties of Personality Responsiveness to Hypnosis

Then there was a question concerning this matter of responsiveness and the outgoing personality. It isn't just a matter of being responsive. You need to look at people, you need to observe people, in order to see how they listen and how they talk to you. The outgoing personality may be responsive; there is a certain intensity of natural, unaffected responsiveness wherein the person behaves as a whole—really listening to you, really talking to you, without an effort to control the environment in any way. And yet you see that responsiveness in a great variety of forms: in the outgoing person, in the withdrawn person, the active, the inactive—in all sorts of personalities.

Individual Trance States

Trance Depth and Locality Determined by Individual Hypnotic Goals: Dental, Psychotherapeutic, and Obstetrical Variations: The Segmented Trance

Another question which I think is an awfully important one is this matter of how to recognize the individual trance states. How do you know if your subject is in a light trance, a medium trance, or a deep trance? The first question you ought to ask yourself is, what is the purpose of the trance being induced? Ted Aston is going to use his hypnosis in dentistry. He wants a type of hypnosis that is oriented about the mouth, and just about the mouth, and that's all. But Bernie Gorton here wants to use his hypnosis on psychiatric patients. So he isn't interested in hypnosis centering around the mouth; he is interested in a hypnosis that governs thinking and emotional behavior. Ted Aston is concerned about pain responses; Bernie Gorton is concerned about emotional reactions. In other words, you use hypnosis in relationship to your patient's needs.

Over and over again I have observed the readiness with which patients spontaneously develop the type of trance that best fits their needs. The dental patient can walk into a dental office and have a nice, oral hypnosis: his legs are out of hypnosis, his hands are out of hypnosis, his body is out of hypnosis, but his mouth and jaw are in hypnosis. And you can have chills run up and down your spine, and when you are cold you can get goose bumps all over your body. But you can also limit those goose bumps to just one arm and just one hand. In hypnosis you have the same opportunity of letting patients respond to the hypnotic situation by doing it locally. Therefore, when you work hypnotically with patients you do not necessarily try to get the same kind of a trance that I use when I want to demonstrate all the varieties of hypnotic phenomena. You may not want the kind of trance wherein you do extensive psychotherapy. The point is that you try to use the kind of hypnosis which will allow your patients to achieve the appropriate hypnotic goals. That's why Dr.

Coulton can have his patients hypnotized from the waist down and deliver their babies while they remain awake from the waist up. Of course they are in a trance state, but they do not need to manifest hypnotic phenomena from the waist up. When I am demonstrating hypnosis comprehensively, I will want all of my subject's body in a trance so that I can utilize any type of hypnotic behavior. So when you use hypnosis, first try to recognize its purpose.

Depotentiating Phobic and Obsessive-Compulsive Behavior

Reframing via Acceptance, Reinterpretation, and Progressive Diminution: "Which Knife to Use?"

[Tape resumes while Erickson is in the middle of reading an audience member's question concerning the treatment of a phobic patient.]
"She would become very agitated whenever she saw a knife or heard people talking about cutting their wrists. She wanted no more shock treatments. She was terrified of shock treatments. She did very well in several sessions, and then one day she called me up in a very agitated state because she was having obsessive thoughts of doing harm to herself by picking up a hatpin and sticking her wrists with it. I immediately saw her and told her how happy this made me, because it was the first evidence of improvement: she had transferred her focus from something lethal such as a knife to something insignificant such as a hatpin. Was this the way to handle this case? It did seem to satisfy her."

One of the reasons patients enter therapy is to receive an acceptance of their particular problem from the therapist. They can't handle the problem themselves yet they have a need to struggle to do something in relationship to their problem. What should you do? *At the first opportunity you ought to accept their behavior in some way, and then you ought to offer them another acceptable interpretation of that behavior.** Yes, that woman did fear cutting her wrists, and she did pick up a hatpin. And although the hatpin is in the same "family" of stabbing instruments as a knife, the hatpin is insignificant whereas the knife is dangerous. *You can reinterpret these situations.* The patient already knew that the hatpin was an insignificant thing. You merely confirmed her choice of a less dangerous means. You allowed her to go through that behavior, but not in such a threatening fashion.

I can cite another example from my own case files. This patient came to me because she was afraid she was going to kill herself with the kitchen butcher knife, and she was also afraid she was going to take that butcher knife and stab her son first. And it was a rather troublesome idea. All day long she kept looking at that butcher knife, thinking about her son, thinking about herself; thinking about how she would appear in the coffin, thinking about how her son would appear in the coffin.

What did I do? After she had described her kitchen to me, I pointed out that there really were quite a number of sharp knives in it. That was simply a fact: there were a number of sharp knives, other than the butcher knife, in her kitchen. So she had another new worry of which knife to use. You know, that's a much better worry than worrying that she *is going* to stab herself, *is going* to stab her son—because now she's got to make a choice of which knife to use before she can carry out those stabbings. And I reiterated that fact of having to choose among a number of kitchen knives. In other words *I just simply reinterpreted the situation by creating a new, legitimate problem. Whenever patients allow you to manipulate their problem situation, try to manipulate it in a way that is acceptable to them.*

> *Eds:* Reframing thus proceeds by reinterpreting the problem situation in a new light: ideas are presented to distract the patient from harmful preoccupations, or, even better,

---

*Eds: Here is another clear expression of the developing concept of reframing.

new variables are introduced to give the patient a sense of control.

Treating Symptomatic Behavior

Symptom Prescription as a Form of Paradoxical Suggestion to Gain Control over Compulsive Movement: 145 Arm Movements Per Minute!

I can think of the patient who had this sort of a behavior [Erickson apparently demonstrates some kind of erratic arm movement]. He moved his arm 135 times in a minute in that fashion, and I couldn't touch him at all. Since I couldn't touch him at all, I increased his arm movements to 145 times a minute. I climbed aboard his boat, so to speak, and increased the symptomatology. But, of course, then I could let it go back to 135 movements per minute, where the patient originally had set it at. Next I moved it up to 140 and dropped it down to 130; up to 135 and down to 125; up to 130 and down to 120. In this way I got a gradual diminution of the symtomatic behavior. But you do not try to fight with your patient. [You participate in the symptomatology by first accepting it, which then opens the possibility of manipulating it out of existence.]

Treating Guilt Indirectly

Imbedding Multiple Levels of Meaning into an Apparently Direct Suggestion: Structuring Implication out of Personal Needs and Values: Paradoxical Suggestion

I had a case of a man who ostensibly came to me for help in correcting his cigarette smoking, but actually he came to me because of overwhelming guilt reactions. He had a frigid wife, a neurotic daughter, and he himself had had many extramarital affairs about which he felt extreme guilt. How would you handle that sort of problem?

I'm going to say something rather shocking, because you are all in the ordinary waking state. I think the way to handle that man's guilt is to teach him to have less guilt reactions about his extramarital affairs. He ought not to have guilt about extramarital affairs. Do you see the transformation there? *He ought to have less guilt about his extramarital affairs... he really ought to have less guilt... he ought to have no guilt at all.* I am seemingly encouraging him to have those extramarital affairs with less guilt, but as he works on my suggestion in accord with the needs of his own personality, *he's going to start lessening the number of his extramarital affairs in order to lessen his guilt.*

You ought to know what goal you have in mind for the patient. In having that guilt reaction, the man was asking me to do something about the correction of his extramarital affairs. But if I had tried to tell him, "Now, cut out those affairs... don't be a bad boy... that's bad behavior," then I would have failed in the therapeutic purpose.

Understanding the Psychodynamics of Cure

The Issue of Underlying Cause in Psychotherapeutic
Problems: Delivering the "Baby" of Mental Health without
Knowing

[In all psychotherapeutic matters there is this issue of underlying cause.] I think that the cause of many problems is very often buried under an accumulation of a lifetime of experience, so that it is very, very difficult to excavate. I'm often reminded of how we can discover a cause in one particular situation, and it is analogous to that need to search into causes in general.

A friend of mine had been married for over 20 years. When she and her husband got married they had both wanted children, and they had set about trying to have children right away. But the years passed and no pregnancies occurred. Extensive examinations were repeated this year, next year, the following year, and so on, and the physicians always came up with the same answer that there was no organic reason to explain her inability to get pregnant.

As the years passed she got more and more discouraged. Finally she developed some symptomatology: her menstrual periods became irregular and finally stopped entirely. Her physician told her that she was going through menopause. After a few months, however, the woman went back to her physician and said, "I'm not in menopause—I'm pregnant!" He laughed at her—he had known her for a long time—and told her that that was just the pseudoscientific thinking of a disappointed woman in menopause. But it turned out that she *was* pregnant.

What was the cause of that 20-year period of sterility? Who is interested? Better to deliver that baby, take care of that baby, and let the mother adjust satisfactorily to her new life. Academically speaking, it would be interesting to know why that woman became pregnant for the first time at the age of 44. *But in many psychiatric cases the real problem is that of delivering the "baby" of mental health to patients so that they can get along satisfactorily; the problem is not that of digging into the past in a frantic endeavor to discover possible causes.*

I had one patient, for example, who had a tremendous fear of red. She just couldn't stand the sight of red. She couldn't go to parties because women wore red clothes, red hats, red flowers, red lipsticks, and red fingernails. She had a most miserable existence.

I don't know what I did for her, and I don't know how I did it. But I visited her in her home after our sessions ended and noticed that she had wallpaper with red cherries on it covering her kitchen walls. Now nobody knows the cause of that terrific red phobia that governed her life so extensively. But she is very happy now. She is very happily married, she has a nice family, and she is very well adjusted socially. I certainly wouldn't try to find out what had caused her original problem. It is in the past. You could try to use hypnosis, and you would probably find some deep-seated cause for her problem located somewhere in the past. But should we try to correct that cause which is so deeply buried, or should we try to correct present-day behavior, present-day living, and the living for tomorrow, the next week, next month, next year?

Trance Induction Methods for Hyperactive Children

The next question is, "Is there any method of induction for children, particularly for nervous, restless, or impatient children?"

The quick, energetic, nervous, excitable, emotionally unstable child can be put into a trance in the same way that you approach the quick, nervous, irritable, excitable adult patient. You try to recognize patients' needs; you try to get their attention, and you try to utilize their behavior. I can't go into this issue right now, but I'll try to go back to it later.

Ideomotor Cues

The Validity of Hand and Head Signaling as a Monitor of Trance Events to Indicate Unconscious Knowledge and Degree of Cooperation: "Those Several Affairs"

Another question concerned the validity of hand motions. A good deal has been said about the procedure of asking the unconscious mind to lift the right hand if the answer is yes, the left hand if the answer is no. The assumption is that the patient's unconscious functions as an entity in itself which can give reliable information. The question asked is how valid is that assumption?

It is only as valid as is your capacity to understand the situation with which you are dealing. A patient came to me and told me that she had a tremendous guilt complex because she had had several affairs over a period of years. And she very willingly gave me the names, dates, places, situations of each of those seven affairs. She was so communicative, so free, so honest and direct in describing all of those experiences, all of her feelings.

But having had some psychiatric experience, I wondered what she would tell me in the trance state. It turned out that in a nice, deep trance state she gave me the same account of the same seven affairs. There were only minor corrections. But her waking account agreed essentially with the trance account.

I had mentioned to her before the possibility of her unconscious giving answers: yes with the right hand or the right index finger, and no with the left hand or the left index finger—just as one could nod the head yes or shake the head no. And I gave that as a simple, incidental explanation, not admonishing her to do it, but just mentioning that it was one of the things that could be done, presumably by some other patient.

She again recounted her affairs in the trance state. She began, "My first affair was in 19—," but her left hand signaled no. I made a mental note of the fact that she had said "my *first* affair" while her hand signaled no.

Next she came to what I think was her fourth affair. She introduced that by saying, "And my next affair," but again her hand signaled no. Three times she signaled no. Once it was her hand that signaled no; once it was her finger that signaled no; and once it was her head signaling no. But she didn't notice any of those movements; she was as unaware as could be. Haven't you ever talked to a bunch of students who were unconsciously nodding or shaking their heads in response to the lecture you were delivering?

In a still later trance I found out that her first affair hadn't occurred at age 17, as she had originally stated. It had occurred at the time of puberty: she had seduced an older man, and had been so overwhelmed with guilt afterwards that she completely repressed it. *That* was her first affair. Then she had forgotten the third or fourth affair, and she had also forgotten the sixth one— repressed them all completely. Yet *I* could ask her, "Did you give me an account of your affairs?; did you give me an account of *all* of your affairs?", and she would say yes. Well, she *had* given me an account of all of her affairs, but, you see, that was all the account she had given me, and that was all of the account she was willing to give me. She was not at all adverse to my knowing that it was an incomplete account—but it was a complete account so far as her willingness to disclose it. In other words, she was saying to me: "You can see what's in this hand, but you can't see what's in that hand."

You ought to bear that in mind when you deal with patients. You can't force them to cooperate, but you can get them to disclose to you how completely or incompletely they are cooperating. I certainly didn't try to force that woman to tell me about those missing accounts until she was ready, and she herself was tremendously surprised to find out about those repressed affairs.

Indirect Techniques for Hypnotic Visualization

Providing a "Multiplicity of Choices" as Progressive, Double-Binding Suggestions to Evoke Sensory-Kinesthetic Memories: The Blackboard Technique

Now the program says I am to discuss indirect techniques. I think all of you have seen me use indirect techniques. One uses indirect techniques by virtue of a willingness to become thoroughly acquainted with all of the other techniques. We have stressed to you the importance of learning the hand levitation technique, the importance of learning the relaxation technique, the importance of learning the coin technique, the importance of learning the blackboard technique, the house-tree-man technique, the imaginary subject technique. Now let us take one of those techniques—the blackboard technique—to see what is really involved in it.

You want to know if the patient is a good visualizer. Perhaps you don't know whether he is, and perhaps he doesn't know either. So you ask him to recall some blackboard. What are you doing when you ask him to remember a certain blackboard? Have you ever put those instruments on the eyelids of a subject to test the behavior of his eyeballs as he is remembering a certain blackboard? What does the subject do with his eyeballs when he starts remembering a certain blackboard? The eyes look from one side to the other side; there is a certain amount of movement of the eyeballs. Those eyeball movements are a part of the process of remembering a certain blackboard.[3]

So you ask your patient to select any one of the blackboards he can recall. He remembers a goodly number of them from his school days, but he takes the one that gives him the most comfortable eyeball movements at the time of remembering. Then you ask him to visualize that blackboard and to note that it has a tray at the bottom—most blackboards have those trays—and that there is chalk in the tray. What do you want him to do? You want him to see the chalk. How do you do that? Your indirect suggestions are tremendously important. There really ought to be a large piece of chalk, a long piece, a medium-sized piece, one or two or three or four small pieces of chalk; perhaps blue chalk and yellow chalk, but chiefly white chalk. In other words, you give a multiplicity of stimuli, a multiplicity of ideas, so that you are certain to hit upon some actual memories belonging to the patient. You are merely evoking past memories: white chalk, blue chalk, yellow chalk. You're going to have that patient follow a visualization technique, and don't you think you ought to get colors into the situation in some way? You're going to have the patient visualize, and how much is going to be visualized? Every possible thing that will fit into the situation. *Therefore you provide a multiplicity of suggestions: the more suggestions that you give, and the more simply you give them, the greater the possibility of getting some of them accepted.* Your task isn't to force a patient to accept suggestions. Your task is to present a sufficient number of suggestions so that he will willingly take this one and take that one.

Next you ask the patient to notice the eraser: is it on the right side or the left side of the tray? Is it right-side up, or backside up, or is it lying on its side? You really don't know, because you yourself aren't visualizing it. And you let the patient know that you don't know. For when you tell a patient that *you* don't know, you are telling the patient at the same time, "But *you* do know"—and that's a tremendously important thing. You give the patient a feeling of certainty and security in his own knowledge that *he* knows, while you do not know.

Now you ask him to pick up a piece of chalk—to visualize himself picking up a piece of chalk—and to inscribe a fairly large circle, a *fairly large* circle. What are you doing? *Large* contradicts *fairly; fairly* contradicts *large.* Therefore you say *fairly large* with two different intonations [*fairly* is spoken softly with a lilt; *large* is spoken in a firm, punctuated tone]. You see, you are offering your subject two different types of suggestions. So now it isn't a question of *is* he going to inscribe a circle; the question is, is it going to be *fairly,* or is it going to be *large?* That's the real question: *how* is he going to inscribe his circle, because you've put it to him that he's going to inscribe a *fairly large* circle. You've made the goal of your suggestion the minor aspect and the quality of your suggestion the major aspect. *But as surely as the patient debates and accepts the question of the quality of the performance, the quantity of the performance, he admits the performance: he has to draw the circle.*

> *Eds:* That is, the subject is double binded into drawing a circle in his imagination: he can debate *how* he will draw the circle, but not *that* he will draw the circle.

What are you really doing when you have the patient visualize himself inscribing that *fairly large* circle? You are asking him to use his judgment; you are asking him to use his memories. What kind of memories are you asking him to use? You are asking him to use the kinesthetic memories of the movement of the hand, the sensory memories of the feeling of chalk in his fingers, the feeling of muscles being used to press chalk against the blackboard, the memories of how the resistance of the blackboard to the chalk feels to the hand and arm, the auditory memories of the sound of chalk being drawn across the blackboard. You are asking him to remember all of that, and he doesn't even know it. *You are asking him to activate a tremendous number of memories.* It isn't just the simple process of saying so many words. *It is the process of getting your patient to do a tremendous number of interrelated things.*

Next you have him step back and look at that blackboard. Is it a debatable question that he is going to step back? No. You have him step back *not* to debate the stepping back, but to "step back and look at the blackboard where you have inscribed that circle." You are asking the patient to make a response requiring kinesthetic memories of muscle movements throughout his life, of sensory memories of the shifting of his weight. What else are you doing? You are getting him to make an increasing number of responses. And so he steps back and looks at the circle. You know, he can't step back to look at that circle without already having drawn the circle. You are confirming the reality of his visualization, and it's awfully important to confirm everything.

How do you confirm the existence of his visualization of the chalk he is picking up?: "You'll probably pick up that center piece of chalk, or the medium-sized piece. But you really don't have to pick up the medium-sized piece. You could even pick up the blue, or the yellow, or that small piece." Again, it is a matter of confirming the existence of the chalk for the subject by the simple process of giving him a multiplicity of choices. He cannot decide *which* piece of chalk to pick up unless there are several pieces right there. And yet you've created a number of pieces, so he picks up your suggestion easily.

Now you ask him to pick up the eraser and erase the blackboard *with a smooth stroke of the eraser.* Why should you want the patient to experience any difficulty about the execution of that visualization? Therefore you put in, "with a *smooth* movement of the eraser." In that way it doesn't become a process of erasing, it becomes a question of the quality of the smoothness of the erasure. And so the patient doesn't dispute whether he is going to erase the blackboard; instead he is involved in the quality of the performance, thereby confirming the performance as something that is going to be done. And all along you are achieving every one of your purposes in an indirect fashion.

Then, naturally you want to know what he sees on the blackboard. And what does he see on the blackboard? You know he should see a smudge from the erasure, and you're going to know very shortly how well he is able to visualize. What do you get? The patient who really can visualize is a little bit shocked to give his reaction. He had said, "No, I see a clean blackboard," and you mention, "Well, don't you see the smudge?" If he makes a rather embarrassed correction then you know he's wondering, "How did I ever fail to see that smudge?", and you also know that you've got a good visualizer. But if he makes a laborious correction, you know then he's not a good visualizer and that you should shift to another technique.

Finally you ask the patient to turn away from the blackboard, *all the way* away from the blackboard. Now I suppose that's a rather silly way of wording it, grammatically speaking. To turn away from the blackboard is one thing. But to turn *all the way* away implies that quality of performance. And the patient is again going to be concerned with the quality of his performance, not with the mere possibility of performance. Therefore he is going to perform as requested.

Individuality of Hypnotherapists

Then you have the patient see a table with flowers on it. Now I personally don't like the way Dr. Secter always agrees with the patient. He will ask, "How many flowers do you see there?" The subject replies, "Two dozen," and Secter says, "That's right, precisely two dozen flowers." I don't like that approach, but then I have a different personality. And I'd like to have all of you be aware of the fact that you ought to disagree with me, just as I disagree with Secter. I disagree with Secter because his approach is wrong for me. But it's right for Secter. *So I want all of you to be willing to disagree with my wording, because it's right for me but it may be wrong for you. When you establish that understanding, you will be free to express your own personalities.*

Easy Trance

Establishing Ideomotor Signaling via Casual Conversation

One of the most important aspects of utilizing hypnosis is teaching patients to go into a trance in the easiest possible fashion. When I see a patient for the first time, and I think he may be a bit difficult to put into a trance, there are certain things I want to be sure of. So I ask a few casual questions, and having asked those casual questions I mention, "Now, you nodded your head yes in reply to that question." That's right, he did, but it's just a casual observation on my part. And later he shook his head no, and I mention that. In other words my indirect, unspoken message to the patient is, "You can answer by nodding your head yes, or you can answer by shaking your head no." I have brought it out in that particular fashion, and I won't need to tell him again during that therapeutic hour that he can answer by nodding his head yes or shaking his head no.

Another Double-Binding Suggestion for Visual Hallucination

Bearing all of that in mind, as the patient turns to look at the table I say, "Perhaps you can see the table there, with the flowers in the middle of it." Now perhaps he can see a table; perhaps he can see the flowers. But the question is, "Perhaps you can see the table there, with the flowers *in the middle of it.*" Again, I make the issue one of quality of performance. So the patient looks at the middle of the table to see if he can see flowers there. And as surely as he accepts the middle of the table, then he accepts the flowers, and so on.

Trance Talking

Now I continue: "And to signify—just to signify—whether you see the flowers in the *middle* of the table, either nod or shake your head." Now how many people grow up with the belief that we should not and cannot talk when we are asleep? And how many hypnotic subjects equate hypnosis with sleep, and therefore cannot talk in a trance state? They mistakenly believe they have to wake up in order to talk. But one of the first things we all have learned from the very beginning of life is that we can be asleep, and we can move in our sleep. So when I get a subject in a trance state, and I want to teach him how to talk in that trance state, I lay the foundation by first teaching him the nodding and shaking of his head in the trance state. You see, everybody knows that we can move when we're asleep.

Once you get the patient to nod or shake his head, you have established a movement of the body that is also a communication. You have taught him to communicate with you. Then you state: "You've nodded your head and that means yes, doesn't it? And it does mean yes, doesn't it?" Here the patient has the opportunity of either nodding his head again, or saying yes. So often patients will answer the question by saying yes. They then have learned verbal communication in the trance state.

Dealing with Resistance in Patients

The Need for Accepting, "Showing," and Utilizing the Patient's Presenting Behavior

With a resistance patient, one of the approaches I use is to get him to manifest that resistance: "I think those flowers are in the middle of the table, but *I don't think you will see them there. You will probably see them over to the left end of the table—I hope it's not the right end of the table."* Now I've got him coming, going, front, back, up, down, all around. I've created that situation: "I don't think you'll see them in the middle." If the patient wants to be really resistant, he can see them right there in the middle. But that's where I want him to see them! [Laughter] Then my statement that he would probably see them at the left end of the table: well, I hope he knows that if he does, it means he's willing to accede in giving me a crumb of encouragement. Or he can defy me still further by seeing those flowers at the right end of the table. What have I done? I've given him plenty of opportunity to express his resistance in order to learn how to function to meet his actual goals in coming into my office.

You ought not lose sight of the fact that the patient comes to you for help, and therefore *you accept his behavior, and you give him plenty of opportunity to show his behavior. You try to help him show his behavior—not to overcome his behavior—but to show his behavior, and you try to use that behavior in a way that will benefit him, not you.* You ought always to keep your hand on the steering wheel of the therapeutic situation and be ready to meet any situation. But you let your patient do all of the behaving in accord with his actual needs. *The beginner in hypnosis often places too much emphasis upon immediately trying to correct the patient's behavior, trying to tell the patient how to behave.*

Enhancing Hallucinations

Paradoxical Suggestions for Response Inhibition; Eliciting Motor Memories and Behavior; Evoking Wonder and Receptivity to the New: "Look in the Other Direction"

Now another approach is to ask the patient, "*About* how long are the stems on those flowers?" It isn't a question of *how long* are they?; it's a question of *about* how long. In other words, "Please don't tell me exactly; please tell me approximately." That means the patient has to *inhibit* his responses regarding the exact length of the stems on the flowers and give you only an approximation. How better to enhance the hallucination of those flowers then by making it necessary for him to inhibit some aspects of those hallucinated flowers? So you are requiring him to do a very, very complicated thing. You are building up his visualizations, and you are utilizing memories of all sorts.

So the patient shows you approximately how long the flowers are. But then you are getting movement. And what do you want your patient to do in therapy? Do you want him to just sit still or lie down, or will it be necessary for that patient to learn how to move about, to shift his body and alter all of his skeletal-muscular behavior? Perhaps if you are a psychiatrist, you will want him to do some automatic writing. Well, the nicest lesson for automatic writing is having him measure, approximately, the length of those hallucinated flowers. And you're getting motor behavior. You have motor behavior memories, and you have actual motor behavior.

After he has measured the length of those flowers and shown you with his hands how long they are, you say: "Well, we can leave the flowers now and look off in the other direction—the *other* direction." What is the *other* direction? You are making use of a word that means exactly what? What is the other direction? You want your patient to have an openness of mind, a readiness to receive ideas, and so you ask him to look off into another direction. And he starts looking and waiting, waiting for you to define that situation. You are the therapist, and he should look to you to define the situation.

Then you say, "You can see a darkness there; you can see a wall with a door—a wall *with a door.*" What's the purpose of that door? That sounds interesting. You've got an openness of the mind, and now what is that door?: "And through that door you can find *another room.*" What have you done? There was the room with the flowers in it, there was the blackboard room, and now there is yet *another room.* And you can populate this room in any way you choose. You can have a chair in there—a red-leather chair, a green-leather chair, a straight-backed chair, a comfortable chair, an uncomfortable chair—any kind of chair you wish.

Creative Utilization of Resistance

Discharging via the Negative, Refocusing via Structured Hallucination, and Resolution via Reassociation: "I Can Do the Gracious Thing"

How would you handle the matter of resistance with this type of hallucination? You can express extreme regret: "I am sorry, but in that room there is a hard, straight-backed chair. It doesn't look comfortable to me, but unfortunately it's the only chair there for you to sit on." What am I doing? I am giving the very, very resistant subject something to direct his antagonism toward, his resistance toward, by making the chair hard and uncomfortable. And as surely as he sees himself sitting down in that chair, he will start experiencing his resistances within himself and not in relationship to me over here. His resistances are going to concern the hardness and the discomfort of the chair.

Then I can be very, very gracious and say, "After you have sat there a few moments, you will begin to feel comfortable." Well, that's what he'd like to do. Who wants to sit in an uncomfortable chair? And I've asked him to please himself, so I've used his resistances to create a situation in which he can please himself. He's coming to me for therapy to please himself, but he's also bringing to me a great deal of resistance. Why not accept that resistance and utilize it? So I have him sit in that uncomfortable chair and watch himself go into a trance as he develops comfort and relaxation. Or, if he wants to be really resistant and I can't get him into that uncomfortable chair, then I can ask him to see someone else sitting in that uncomfortable chair. And he isn't going to like the discomfort of the other person sitting in that chair. I'm using his resistance, but then I can do the gracious thing of letting that hallucinated subject sit in that uncomfortable chair and feel very, very comfortable. And he, too, is wishing that that hallucinated subject were sitting in a comfortable chair, and he is thereby led to reject his own resistance.

PART IV

SPECIAL STATES OF AWARENESS AND RECEPTIVITY*

The Nature of Hypnosis

Receptivity to Ideas and Recognition of Inherent Values: Recalling a Breakfast Forty-Five Years Ago

In discussing hypnosis in medicine, I would like to present it first from a general point of view. Then I will call upon some volunteer subjects to present the various hypnotic phenomena, and to illustrate some of the possible uses.

I'm going to be rather informal in my presentation. As I said, I'm simply going to discuss hypnosis in general. As a preliminary to any discussion, I would like to define *hypnosis as a state of special awareness characterized by a receptiveness to ideas*. That receptiveness allows the person to examine the new ideas for their inherent worth. Once the ideas have been examined, the subject is then at liberty to accept or reject them. If the ideas are accepted, the subject then responds to those ideas in accordance with their inherent worth.

Perhaps the best way to illustrate my point is with this example. If you were to ask a 50-year-old man, "What did you eat for breakfast on your fifth birthday?; what did you wear?; on which side of the table did you sit?," his immediate response is likely to be, "Why, that was 45 years ago!" Indeed, who would

*Lecture given before The American Society of Clinical Hypnosis in Youngstown, Ohio, 1959.

bother to remember what he had eaten for breakfast 45 years ago? Who would bother to remember something so unimportant as on which side of the table he had sat?

But, you see, there is actually a great deal of inherent worth in those questions, which one would recognize in the hypnotic trance state. Why? Because, again, *it is a state of special awareness, of special receptiveness to ideas, of special willingness to examine ideas for their inherent values.* The 50-year-old man in the trance state [would immediately begin to revive his memories in order to answer the question.] Why? He would recognize that his fifth birthday had been a culmination of a lifetime of experience. After all, it had been his first and only fifth birthday. He had felt tremendously important on that particular day, even though at the time he didn't quite understand why. He just knew it was important: it had culminated five years of his life—in fact, it had culminated his entire lifetime. So it was an outstanding event. And everything that had happened on that particular day was eventful, whether it was what he had worn, or on which side of the table he had sat.

So the 50-year-old man in the trance state will examine that idea, that question, in terms of its actual, inherent values. He will recognize, "Yes, I've had many breakfasts, many birthdays. I had my fortieth birthday, and my thirtieth birthday; my twentieth, my fifteenth, my tenth, and my fifth. And when I was 5 years old, I lived at such-and-such a place, and my brother was so many years old; we ate these things, we ate those things; these were the things I liked as a child, [these were the things I didn't like]."

In other words he would very, very promptly build up a full recollection of the food he had eaten for breakfast on his fifth birthday, of the clothes he had worn, of where he had sat at the table. Willingly he would revive those memories and be able to report them. He would not make the ordinary conscious response of dismissing the question as irrelevant, just because it referred to events some 45 years ago. He would not respond, "Why, who would bother to remember all of those irrelevant and impertinent references and evaluations?!" He would recognize they were neither irrelevant nor impertinent.

The Unconscious Mind in Hypnosis

Hypnotic and Dream Processes Utilizing and Integrating Previous Experiential Learnings with Current External Realities

The next thing I want to point out to you is this: in hypnosis you use the *unconscious mind*. I'm not going to try to define *unconscious mind* for you, because it's too familiar a concept—it's too convenient a concept—for me to bother about defining. But we know that in ordinary, everyday, conscious thinking, we have a tendency to devote a large part of it to orienting ourselves to our immediate surroundings. For example, at the present time you are listening to me, you are also aware of the fact that somebody is sitting to the left of you, to the right of you, behind you, and in front of you; you are aware of the fact that I am holding a microphone in my hands, that I'm sitting down, that there are lights in the ceiling, that there is a clock above my head—all of those irrelevant considerations. Why? Because we need to keep consciously in touch with our surroundings.

Our hypnotic thinking, however, is that of the unconscious mind; we give our attention solely to a particular idea, to a particular thought of value or significance in the immediate situation. In that kind of thinking, you pay no attention to irrelevant surroundings, because they aren't a part of the situation. In the hypnotic trance, you would listen to me; and you would merely listen to the ideas that I presented. It wouldn't be necessary for you to include in your awareness the perceptions that I was sitting down, that I was in front of you, that I was holding a microphone in my hand, that I was sitting next to the table, and so forth. You would give your full, conscious attention solely and simply to the ideas being presented.

The type of thinking used in hypnosis is the type of thinking that you use in your nighttime dreaming. You can be sound asleep in bed, resting very comfortably at the physiological level, yet be dreaming that a very treasured friend is visiting you. You take your friend and go out into the backyard. You talk to the friend, you show him the flowers in your garden, you listen to the birds; your friend speaks to you, and you speak to your friend. Now that dream can be utterly and completely vivid and real, as if your friend and you were standing in your garden, "in the flesh." You see, in your nighttime dreaming you are employing memories, ideas, emotions, and images of all sorts—kinesthetic memories and images, auditory images, visual images—all sorts of learnings that constitute your whole life's experience. You simply revivify all of those learnings to effect the immediate mental picture that you are developing in the dream. That is exactly what you do in hypnosis: you take ideas, thoughts, memories, and images of all sorts.

In your nighttime dreaming you can turn over in bed, which happens to be against the bedroom wall, and rest your back against the wall. Meanwhile, in your dream of being in the garden, that is the moment you sit down in the garden chair and lean back against it. *In the process of dreaming, you translate the stimuli of external reality into the dream content that you are experiencing. In hypnosis, you have that same opportunity of using abstract memories and ideas, as well as utilizing stimulation from external reality.* That is one of the reasons why hypnosis is tremendously valuable in the practice of medicine and dentistry: you have the opportunity of teaching patients how to select out of their current reality the things that they can use; how to select out of their total lifetime experiences the things they can use in their particular situations. *All hypnotic phenomena are based upon normal experiences and normal behaviors, which are then extended and utilized in a controlled and directed manner.*

Catalepsy and Amnesia

Hypnotic Phenomena as Normal Patterns of Behavior
Organized for Intentional Therapeutic Purposes

I'll give you some examples to illustrate. Later I'll demonstrate the phenomenon of catalepsy in which a hand can be lifted up (like this), and it will remain indefinitely in that position. Psychology laboratory experiments have demonstrated that a hand can remain in that type of position for as long as four hours without appreciable, measurable fatigue. But we see the same phenomenon in everyday, normal life—we just don't recognize it. How do you manage to hold your head upright all day long, except through the balanced muscle tonicity of the muscles in your neck? You do that all day long, but just as surely as you begin to feel tired, your head may sag to one side or the other; it may come to rest on your chest; or it may actually tilt backward. Each of us has his own particular pattern of responding to fatigue, but the point is that the balanced muscle tonicity of catalepsy is something that also characterizes ordinary everyday life.

Another hypnotic phenomenon is this matter of amnesia, whereby you can forget things very quickly. What types of things can you forget in the trance state? You can forget names, and you can forget pain. [But you forget names and pain in everyday ordinary life as well.] You are introduced to a person; you shake hands while repeating the name; yet scarcely a second after you've repeated the name, you start scratching your head and wondering, "Now what was his name? I really should remember!" And you casually look around the room, hoping that somebody will call that person by name. That way, you won't have to be embarrassed by asking to be told again—just to discover that once again you've instantly forgotten it.

So, you see, forgetting things is a matter of everyday experience. Forgetting pain is also a matter of everyday experience. Did you ever go into a suspense movie with a headache or a toothache, and then not remember until the next day that you had had a toothache, or a headache? What happened to your toothache or your headache; what happened to your aching foot after you got absorbed in the suspense movie? It was a plain matter of a dissociation, a distraction. *All hypnotic phenomena are made up of normal everyday patterns of behavior, organized to serve intentional purposes for the patient.*

The Everyday Basis of Hypnotic Phenomena

Selection and Utilization of Lifetime Learnings for Body Anesthesias and Hypnotic Deafness

Now there is another general point that I want to make about hypnosis so that you can better understand it, and so that you can better appreciate its applications in medicine and dentistry.

Every year a baby starts from scratch to learn a great number of different things. The baby plays with its toes, its knees, its ankles, with all parts of its body; its fingers, its hair, its nose, its eyes, its ears, its mouth, and so on, in an effort to understand the total body configuration. And that body is constantly changing in size, so the baby has to learn again and again.

In a lifetime of experience, what are the things that we actually learn about our bodies? You'll hear the surgeon telling the anesthesiologist that you can't really expect to produce a hypnotic anesthesia that can withstand a laparotomy.* And yet you *can* produce that kind of an anesthesia, psychologically. How is it done? By utilizing the tremendous amount of learning you have acquired during your lifetime of experience in developing anesthesias throughout your entire body. For example, as you sit and listen to me now, you've forgotten the shoes on your feet... and now you can feel them; you've forgotten the glasses on your nose... and now you can feel them; you've forgotten the collar around your neck... and now you can feel it; you've forgotten the sleeves on your arms, and so forth.

You listen to an entertaining lecture, and you forget about the hardness of the chairs. But if it happens to be a very boring lecture, your chair feels so utterly uncomfortable. You sense those things. We've all had tremendous experience in developing anesthesias in all parts of our bodies.

You wonder about hypnotic deafness, and yet you've had the

---

*Editors' Note: A *laparotomy* is a procedure usually reserved for exploratory operations, involving an incision of the abdominal wall.

experience of being so absorbed in reading a book that you don't hear your wife speak to you. Ten minutes later you say, "Oh! Did you say something?" You didn't really hear her at the time; you just had a vague awareness that there may have been a stimulation. So throughout your life you've been learning all of these things that can be selected and utilized.

The Control and Alteration of Physiological Functioning

Utilizing Unconscious Body Learnings: An Experimental Hypnotic Approach to Raynaud's Disease via a Posthypnotic Trance

There is another point I want to make about the body's learnings—about this matter of learning from the experience of living. If I were to ask any one of you in ordinary everyday experience to control your blood vessels, alter your blood pressure, contract your veins, arteries or capillaries, you would look at me rather blankly. How would you really go about it? Yet your total body experience is such that a small word can make you turn red with embarrassment or white with anger; it can raise your blood pressure some 20 points. The mere utterance of a single word! We've all had that kind of experience repeatedly. Part of life involves recording all of those experiences in your unconscious mind, and in hypnosis you're dealing with the unconscious mind. So you present ideas of that inner control to the patient in such a fashion that the patient receives the ideas and translates them into action.

I can think of a case I encountered that well illustrates what I mean. A patient came into my office suffering from Raynaud's Disease. For the benefit of those who don't know what Raynaud's Disease is, it is a neurological disease, a vascular disease, in which the tips of the fingers turn white due to poor circulation. It's a very, very painful disease, especially when the fingers start ulcerating. Then it becomes unbearable pain.

This patient began with the statement that for the past ten years she had been suffering from ulceration of her fingers—such painful ulcerations that she had not slept longer than two continuous hours in ten years. She would fall asleep from exhaustion, sleep for an hour, or an hour-and-a-half, or possibly two hours; then rouse up, pace the floor, and go back to bed. She already had suffered the amputation of one finger to correct that painful ulceration, and she was anticipating losing other fingers. She wanted to know if hypnosis could do anything for her. Now I hadn't really had any experience in the treatment of that particular disease, and I just didn't know whether or not I could help her. But I did have the feeling that this 50-year-old woman had had enough lifetime experience with her total body to be able to correct her physical condition unconsciously—or, at the very least, alleviate some of the pain.

I put her in a trance. After I had her in the trance, I explained to her that her unconscious mind could organize all of her experiential learnings, and it could organize them very thoroughly. She had come into my office that morning; throughout the rest of the day, her unconscious mind would be sifting through her total body learnings. That night at bedtime (which was around a quarter before eleven) she was to sit down in a chair, recall the trance she had experienced in my office, go into another deep trance, and then let her unconscious mind take all the learnings it had been reviewing during the day and apply them in such a way as to provide her with a good night's sleep.

I didn't know what that woman was going to do. I told her to call me up at 11:30, or thereabouts, to let me know what her unconscious had decided was the right therapy for her. At 11:30 the woman called me up and said: "I'm sitting in a chair. [Her voice was quavering.] I'm scared... I'm awful scared... I'm just scared to death. I'm so weak that I can hardly stand up, and I'm so tired that it's hard even to talk."

"What happened in the trance?" I asked.

"I went into a trance just the way you taught me," she answered. "All of a sudden I began to get awfully cold. I got colder and colder, just like I used to get cold in the wintertime when I lived in northern Minnesota. I shivered and trembled, and my teeth chattered for at least ten minutes. It was the coldest I had ever been in my life. It was horrible, suffering like that from the cold. Then all of a sudden the cold started to leave me and I began to feel very warm and very hot all over."

Of course, I recognized what she was talking about from my experience in Wisconsin: you chill your ears, you get them awfully cold, and then as they warm up they feel bone hot. In the same way, her entire body felt as if it were burning up. There was a tremendous amount of vascular dilatation all over her body, and she felt very, very weak. As she described that weak feeling to me, I asked her if she didn't mean that she felt tremendously relaxed. She said she did. I told her to go to bed and give me a telephone call in the morning. She went to bed immediately.

At eight o'clock that morning she phoned me to report: "I'm so surprised. I could scarcely crawl into bed I was so relaxed, and I must have fallen asleep immediately. I didn't wake up until just a couple of minutes ago, so I thought I'd call you right away. Maybe my unconscious does know how to handle the pain of Raynaud's Disease."

Raynaud's Disease is a neurological vascular disease involving a sensitized reaction to cold, so she had brought about a tremendous alteration in the circulation of her blood. From her evening report, I now knew what suggestions to give her. That day I explained to her: "You know, you really don't need to get cold all over. You don't need to chatter your teeth for ten minutes, and you don't need to shiver. Just get cold enough so that you can get warm enough at bedtime to relax completely, go right to sleep, and sleep comfortably throughout the night."

Now the woman has her pain during the day, but she is progressing a great deal. The ulceration has been arrested, and one of the ulcers is healing slightly, very slowly. She is no longer anticipating going back to the Mayo Clinic, nor having another finger, or another couple of fingers, amputated. She is getting between six to eight hours of sleep every night, after ten years of not being able to sleep more than two continuous hours.

The Unconscious Alteration of Physiological Functioning

Common Everyday Examples Utilizing Body Learnings

I used this case to illustrate my point that *in hypnosis the unconscious mind searches through the total experiential learnings of the body and organizes them* in such a way that you, as the anesthesiologist, can tell the patient to develop an anesthesia that can withstand a laparotomy. You, as the surgeon, can tell the patient: "After this operation, I'd really like to have you feel rested, and comfortable, and at ease post-operatively. I'd like to have you feel comfortable throughout the body. And you will make a rapid and easy recovery." You, as the obstetrician, can tell the obstetrical patient how to behave and how to experience certain procedures [in a positive and comfortable way].

You also can do what that English physician did when he was confronted with the problem of grafting skin from his patient's leg to the abdomen (or was it from the abdomen to the leg?—I don't remember). The question was, should he put his patient in a cast to keep him in the horribly awkward position for the three weeks' time that would be required if the skin graft were to take hold properly? Well, that English physician decided that he would use the balanced muscle tonicity of catalepsy instead of that cast. So he took his badly burned patient and put him into that horribly awkward position, impressing upon the patient that he would maintain that position, whether he was awake or asleep, until the skin grafts took hold. And the patient did maintain that horribly awkward position, and he did it without developing any pressure sores as a result of a cast (because there was no cast!), and without experiencing any tissue constriction from bandages (because there were no bandages!).

Perhaps I'd better add one more everyday experience. The mother can be exceedingly tired, very, very tired, and she also can be very worried about the baby. She can be so exhausted that she falls into a deep sleep the minute her head hits the pillow. But let that baby utter one single little yip, and she is wide awake. Otherwise, the house could fall apart, an earthquake could occur, and so on, and she would sleep through it all.

In the same way, you can cue patients hypnotically so that they select out of their present external stimuli the things that are requisite to govern their behavior.

In applying all of these ideas to individual patients, there are any number of experiences which you yourselves have already had. For example, as medical or dental students you all had the experience of discovering how tremendously you could alter your physiological behavior. How many times did you walk into a classroom very happily, only to hear the professor (who got up on the wrong side of the bed that morning) announce that he was going to spring a written quiz on you? Now, I don't know how it was with your medical school class, but I know what happened in my medical school class under those circumstances. We divided into two groups immediately: there was the diarrhetic group, and then there was the peristaltic group. [Laughter] And how does that announcement so tremendously alter the physiological functioning of otherwise hearty and healthy medical students? But it does.

Now when you encounter that businessman who is guilty of completely imaginary worries, all located in his head, maybe you can better understand how it is possible for those purely imaginary worries to put holes into his gastric mucosa; or to understand how, when he gets out of that business with a huge profit and goes into some other kind of business (because he couldn't take *that* particular business—he got stomach ulcers), and the new business is going along very nicely and making a reasonable profit, he now gets mucosa colitis! Why? Because he's still got all those purely imaginary worries. How did he manage to [behave physiologically] in those ways? Well, *we do have the capacity of translating various aspects of our psychological experience into physiological functioning—and also into physiological malfunctioning.*

Then we can recall those student days when we got sent a box of fudge. We watched the postman come down the street carrying a package; we discovered that the package was for us; we opened it and found the nice, homemade fudge; and our mouths watered at the sight of it. When that postman came down the street the very next day, carrying an appetizing-looking specimen under his arm, as soon as we saw him our salivary glands—

which are completely without visual powers—immediately started to salivate. Why? Because we had been conditioned by that one single experience.

You see what a tremendous amount of physiological learning, physical learning, and functional learning goes on in the body throughout a lifetime of experience. We utilize hypnosis as a means of creating in our patients an attentiveness in ideas, a fixation on a particular idea; then we allow them to accept that idea, to examine it, and having examined it for its actual inherent value, to deal with it in terms of their total learnings.

DEMONSTRATION

Utilizing Humor to Establish Comfortable, Human Relationships in Hypnosis

Now I think I've given a sufficiently general account of body learnings and experiential learnings. Perhaps the best way to proceed at this point is to illustrate the various hypnotic phenomena and to discuss them as they are demonstrated. Dr. Kay Thompson has been introduced to you previously, and I've used Dr. Thompson before as a subject.

E: Will you come up here please? [Subject is heard walking toward the front.] Do you mind standing up please?

S: I don't mind.

E: You don't mind. Would you come closer to...* [Laughter] Now my reason for that is this [having her stand closer] ... but those in the back of the room didn't have much chance to see what was going on, and I'd like to have you see the demonstration. So, Kay, if you don't mind we can do the demonstration standing. All right. Now, I used you once be-

---

**Editors' Note:* Ellipsis points indicate inaudible material lost in the recording.

234

fore. Was it Baltimore? It was. Will you step closer please...
Had you ever been in a deep trance?

S: Not since I had a baby.

E: We used a light-to-medium trance, isn't that right?
And you volunteered in a halfhearted fashion?

S: I didn't know I was going to volunteer. [Laughter]

E: You didn't know you were going to volunteer, and you didn't know you were going to go into a deep trance. And yet you were perfectly willing to cooperate with me. Tell me, what do you think about this audience?

S: They are fascinating.

E: They are fascinating. Why? Because they are predominantly men? [Laughter]

What I am trying to impress upon you with this flippancy is the following: you do not have to wear a tuxedo, and a starched shirt, and a tall silk hat, and show a lot of stuffed dignity. You want to deal with patients on a purely human level, at a level of good, personal interrelationship. You ought not intimidate or terrify your patients. You ought to let them know that you've got a good, human interest in them.

A Conversational Hypnotic Induction

"Wider Awake" and Confusing Tonal Reversals as Paradoxical Suggestions for Indirect Hypnotic Induction; Involuntary Eye Closure as Ratification of Trance; The Essence of Therapeutic Hypnosis

E: ... How extensively do you use hypnosis in your practice?

S: Like a very expensive catcher's mitt. I use it when I think it is called for.

E: That's right. And sometimes when you are dealing with patients, do you use the hypnotic techniques rather than a formal hypnotic trance?

S: Quite often.

E: That is, you can use your hypnosis, or you can use hypnotic techniques. Now, Kay, you are staying out of the trance, aren't you?

S: I'm trying! [Laughter]

E: But you feel that you are out of the trance?

S: So far.

E: So far. [Much laughter] So far... Now, instead of trying to show you a formal trance induction, I am merely going to talk to Kay, and talk to you. Kay, are you still out of the trance?

S: I think so.

E: Well, *stay wide awake, will you?* [Voice is soft and earnest.] *Wider awake, wider awake* [spoken in the soft, hypnotic tones normally used for "deeper asleep"—faint, muffled chuckling from the audience]. *That's right. Wider awake. And you will stay wider awake, won't you?*

S: I think so.

E: You think so. And do you know whether or not you are in a trance?

S: *I'm not sure.*

E: You're not sure. Is there anybody here you would like to ask if you're in a trance?

S: You.

E: Will you take my word for it?

S: Uh-huh.

E: You will? Well, I'll tell you what. Let's take your word for it. *If your eyes close involuntarily, that will signify that you are in a trance.* [Pause] Do you think you're in a trance?

S: Uh-huh.

E: But you didn't really know for a certainty until you waited for your eyes to close—to see if they would close involuntarily. Isn't that right?

S: ... It startled me.

E: **It startled you because your eyes closed rather abruptly.**

Now I'm going to ask you to note what Kay says and how she says it, because "it startled" her. And Kay has done a lot of hypnosis; she has used it, she has had previous experience with it, and yet it startled her to see how quickly her unconscious mind could take over.

> Eds: This is a highly typical illustration of Erickson's informal, indirect, "conversational" hypnotic induction. Here he uses paradoxical suggestions and subtle, sudden reversals to induce confusion, uncertainty, and not knowing in the modern, rational mind. This type of approach is especially useful for the modern, highly educated conscious mind that seeks hypnotic experience as a means of breaking out of its learned limitations.[1]
>
> Kay Thompson, D.D.S., is one of Erickson's most outstanding students, and is herself an experienced hypnotic operator and subject. Yet even she responds with an "I'm not sure" to the question of whether or not she is in trance after Erickson exposes her to the paradoxical suggestion, "Stay wide awake." Of course, "Stay wide awake" paradoxically implies, "Go into trance" to a sophisticated subject. Erickson then reinforces the confusion of paradox by

urging, "wider awake, wider awake," spoken in the soft, earnest, hypnotic tones normally used for "deeper asleep" suggestions. He thus uses the covert implication of his tonal cues to reverse the overt meaning of his spoken words.

Next Erickson ratifies the presence of trance by facilitating an abrupt, involuntary eye closure which Kay experiences as startling proof of her trance state. Notice that Erickson did not tell her or command her to close her eyes. Such a direct suggestion would prove nothing to a modern, rational mind seeking proof of the existence of an altered state through involuntary or non-intentional behavior. Erickson's permissive contingent suggestion, "If your eyes close involuntarily, that will signify you are in trance," gives the subject's unconscious an opportunity to validate the presence of an altered state via the involuntary behavior that is suggested. He is thus facilitating (guiding, structuring, directing, controlling) the process, but in a way that allows the subject's unconscious to make the crucial choice.

This is the paradoxical essence of the art of modern therapeutic hypnosis: *How to facilitate creative processes in a focused and directive manner while permitting the patient's own individuality to make the important therapeutic choices.*

Trance Motivation

An Inward Focus Based on Interest in One's Own Unconscious Behaviors

E: Are your arms comfortable, Kay?

S: Yes.

E: Was I talking to anybody?

S: [Long pause] Yes [spoken in a soft, exhaling manner].

E: Why do you say yes?

S: Because I knew I was hearing your voice, but I haven't been paying much attention.

E: She knows she was hearing a voice, but she wasn't paying attention.

You see, she is in a trance because she is primarily interested in doing the things that come out of her own unconscious behavior. And it really isn't important for her to pay attention to what I say to you, because you as a group are external to her interest. You are really not important to her.

E: Was I speaking again, Kay?

S: [Pause] Yes [spoken in a whisper].

E: ... In other words, whatever I say now to you is relatively unimportant. And you really don't need to listen, do you Kay?

S: [No response.]

E: And you don't need to listen, do you?

S: No [soft, drawn out].

E: [Silence; very long pause before he addresses the audience.]

Faked Versus Hypnotic Responses

Differentiating by Demonstration of Hand and Arm Catalepsy for Trance Deepening

Now you touch the hand, and you indicate by the nature of your touch that you want it to go down. I could call for any volunteer here today who has never been in a hypnotic trance and ask him to fake that sort of thing. Then I could touch his hand, and this is exactly what would happen with anybody who tries to fake a catalepsy. I'll show you. [Pause as Erickson demonstrates] The hand doesn't stop going down when you cease the pressure, because the person begins to understand that you want the hand to go down and so completes the movement. But Kay, being in a trance, only responds to the specific stimulus that I give. I think this matter of giving stimuli and knowing exactly how you are giving it is one of the important points for you to learn.[2] Now I am going to lift Kay's arm, and I am going to try to illustrate to you this particular approach. [Long pause]

Now what I do is this. Without any noticeable additional pressure, I press down with this finger using this thumb... I am going to fixate your attention on this one idea of being increasingly alert, increasingly alert to this one idea of being awake, which means alert. And so Kay is exceedingly alert to whatever it is I say, exceedingly responsive to whatever I say, and the unimportance of this entire room develops. And at the present time I don't even know whether Kay remembers where she is, and I am going to inquire.

Literalism as a Trance Indicator

Responding to Exact Stimuli Presented as an Unconscious, Uncritical Process

E: Kay, where are you?

S: [Pause] On the platform.

E: She's on the platform. Where is the platform?

S: In an auditorium.

E: In an auditorium. Now where is the auditorium?

S: [Pause] In a hospital.

E: And where is the hospital?

S: [Pause] I don't know.

E: You don't know.

... All of you know where this hospital is located, and all of you are thinking it is in Youngstown, Ohio, or the environs of Youngstown. So why doesn't Kay know that she came here tonight? She isn't stupid. Why doesn't she know she is in Youngstown? But the truth is, where is this hospital? I don't know, because a patient in a trance listens to you and understands exactly what you say. Where is this hospital? It is on a street!

E: Is this hospital on a street, Kay?

S: It is surrounded by streets.

E: It is surrounded by streets.

Now you see she corrected me ... It really isn't *on* a street—a street is a thoroughfare. But it is *surrounded* by streets! Kay just mentions where it is because she doesn't know the names of the streets that surround it.

E: What city is it in, Kay?

S: Youngstown.

E: Youngstown.

You have to ask her specific questions. Now that I've introduced you to these various aspects of hypnosis, you ought to be willing to check out each one of these phenomenon so that you can recognize them in a patient.

Eds: Erickson is demonstrating the phenomenon of literalism wherein the subject in trance tends to respond in a very exact manner to questions. Testing for literalism was one of Erickson's favorite methods of indirectly assessing the presence of a trance state.[3] Future researchers might explore the hypothesis that hypnotic phenomena in general are actually all different manifestations of literalness wherein subjects respond to the exact meaning of suggestions without the mediating influence of reflective thinking.

Please note that although Erickson continued the demonstration at this point, we have ended the Youngstown lecture here because of the poor quality of the audio tape from which we were working. Anyone in possession of a clear tape of this lecture is encouraged to send a copy of it to:

The Milton H. Erickson Foundation
3606 North 24th Street
Phoenix, Arizona 85016

PART V

LIFE REFRAMING

Facilitating Potentials in a Young Photographer*

Introduction

The following transcript of Erickson's work with a young photographer was typical of the type of hypnotherapeutic demonstrations conducted in the early days of The American Society of Clinical Hypnosis. Erickson was introduced to the subject, a young photographer with a stuttering problem, by Dr. H who was the subject's therapist. From the transcript it is evident that they had had a breakfast meeting together a short time before the demonstration was to take place. This gave Erickson a brief, informal period to assess the subject and learn a few things about him that could be used to facilitate the hypnotherapeutic work.

This transcript is an unusually revealing example of Erickson's general approach to trance induction and the facilitation of unconscious potentials. Since the first portion of the audio tape was fairly clear, it is being made available with this volume so that the reader can gain some impression of Erickson's use of vocal cues and pauses for their psychodynamic effects. So intricate is this transcript, however, that we, the editors, could not resist the temptation to provide an organizing commentary as a guide to some of the hypnotherapeutic processes that were most

---

*Audio cassette of this transcript accompanies the volume. Date and location are unknown.

obvious to us. These commentaries, of course, reflect our personal perceptions and learned limitations. They are offered only as heuristics to stimulate the reader's own observations and thinking about the many levels of communication and meaning in the transcript. Erickson would be very poorly served, indeed, if his work was to be constrained to the procrustean bed of the editors' perception of him. The reader is thus encouraged to reframe this transcript in any other way that brings out fresh insights unique to the reader's own way of perceiving, understanding, and doing.

The material of this presentation seemed to divide itself naturally into four sections:

I. Naturalistic Approaches to Trance Induction
II. Evoking Unconscious Potentials
III. Facilitating Active Trance Work
IV. Reframing, Posthypnotic Suggestion, and Trance Ratification

This division, of course, is artificial and is presented here only for didactic purposes. Earlier and equally arbitrary outlines of Erickson's work divided it into five stages[1] and three stages.[2] The careful student will recognize that however the pie is cut, the underlying hypnotherapeutic process is the same. We have summarized each part with a diagram of the associative networks of mutually supportive indirect suggestions and approaches Erickson used to evoke and facilitate "that reassociation and reorganization of ideas, understandings, and memories so essential for an actual cure."

SECTION I:

NATURALISTIC APPROACHES TO TRANCE INDUCTION

"Mind Wandering"

A Naturalistic Approach to Trance Induction: Utilizing an Associative Network of Mutually Reinforcing Ideodynamic Processes

E: *Of course you can be interested consciously in what I say, but even though you may be intensely interested consciously, I would like to have you appreciate the fact that you are infinitely more interested on an unconscious level. And consciously you can just relax; you can close your eyes and let your mind wander at will, from my words, to thoughts of... Dr. H, to thoughts of the water, to thoughts of your daily work, to thoughts of what you had for breakfast today— every wandering thought that comes into your mind. There should be no effort on your part to try to listen to me, no effort whatsoever.*

Ernest Rossi (ER): Erickson begins with the obvious truism, "Of course you can be interested consciously in what I say." Most people are interested in what the therapist is going to say to initiate hypnosis. An expression of this obvious fact causes the subject to make an inner response of yes to this first phrase, and tends to open a *yes set* to accept the mildly surprising second half of the sentence containing the really important suggestion: "but even though you may be intensely interested consciously, I would like to have you appreciate the fact that *you are infinitely more interested on an unconscious level.*" Thus while accepting the conscious mind's interest, Erickson actually utilizes this interest to reinforce the more important focus on the activation of an unconscious level.

Having thus focused interest on the unconscious, Erickson then dismisses and depotentiates the conscious mind with his next casual remark, "And *consciously you can relax;* you can close your eyes and *let your mind wander* at will." This all sounds so easy and permissive, yet very potent *ideodynamic* processes are being set in motion. These *ideas* actually activate major psychophysiological *dynamics* for facilitating trance. Simply *closing the eyes* results in an increase in the resting alpha rhythm of the cerebral cortex; that is, the *central nervous system* is shifted toward a resting inner focus. *Relaxing* facilitates the parasympathetic or resting processes of the *autonomic nervous system*. Thus in one sentence the two major psychophysiological systems regulating consciousness and behavior are nudged in tandem toward a quietly receptive mode. Together with mind wandering they become an ideodynamic invitation for the subject to experience the most natural form of trance available to everyone: the common everyday trance that we all experience throughout the day when we "take-a-break" and let our minds wander. We have speculated previously that mind wandering is an expression of the natural, psychophysiological relaxation rhythm[3] wherein we are predisposed throughout the day (approximately every 90 minutes) to periods of right–hemispheric and parasympathetic activity. At night, dreaming (REM sleep) takes place during these recurrent cycles.

Erickson ends with: "... from my words to ... every wandering thought that comes into your mind. There should be no effort on your part to try to listen to me, no effort whatsoever." What a profound turnabout has taken place in just a few, well-tuned sentences! Let us review it as a three-stage process:

(1) In the first part of the first sentence the subject's obvious conscious interest was acknowledged and accepted;

(2) This conscious interest was then utilized to focus attention on the unconscious, now activated by a mention of one of its most natural and commonly experienced indicators—the mind wandering; and

(3) With the unconscious thus activated, Erickson was then able to dismiss and depotentiate conscious intentionality with "There should be no effort on your part to try to listen to me, no effort whatsoever."

From an acknowledged focus of high conscious interest and a yes set, to an activation of the unconscious mind and a dismissal of conscious effort and intentionality—trance is facilitated with this associative network of three or four mutually reinforcing ideodynamic processes that could be accepted easily by anyone.

This does not mean that the conscious mind is extinguished. On the contrary, the conscious mind is usually present with varying degrees of focus and continuity as a calm witness[4] to some of the inner experiences that are taking place during trance. When Erickson says, "There should be *no effort* on your part to try," he is reinforcing *the lack of conscious intentionality* that is so characteristic of hypnotic responsiveness. The conscious mind may observe, but it more or less stands aside while the unconscious follows its own natural autonomous tendencies—some of which may be to receive and utilize in its own way a few suggestions from the therapist.

"Opening Flower" Metaphor

Beginning the Therapeutic Associational Network by Accessing the Unconscious Mind

E: *Just as you watch a flower open, you can sit and watch without making any effort of your own.* **In exactly the same way you let your unconscious mind open and do its own thinking, its own feeling, without any effort whatsoever on**

your part. All you need to know is that your unconscious mind does exist; it is within you; *it is part of you that you do not really know, but which knows a tremendous amount about you.*

ER: Just as one can quietly sit and watch a flower open, so one can let the unconscious mind open and pursue its course without any effort by the internal observer. This "opening flower" metaphor is a visually poetic image, particularly appropriate for a young, creatively oriented person with an interest in photography. Who among us has not seen and admired the many film images of an opening flower? This utilization of a photographer's interest in the visual maintains the *yes set* to reinforce further the activation of the unconscious. This activation continues and is stabilized with a developing associational network of ideas about the unconscious mind that is beginning to build the foundation of a therapeutic belief system: the unconscious can do the needed healing by using its own natural processes. This is emphasized in the final phrases, "it is a part of you that you do not really know, but which knows a tremendous amount about you." Thus this section ends with a haunting overview of the potency of the unconscious with its ability to cure—since it indeed "knows a tremendous amount about you."

Facilitating Human Potentials

Associating the Patient's Highest Potentials with the Autonomous Activity of the Unconscious; Transference as a Mediator of Highest Potentials

E: *At the breakfast table you mentioned the matter of portrait photographs, and the expressiveness of them, and the oversight of them; and yet your unconscious knows when and how and why you developed that interest.* **You've spoken about your photographic hobby. You have it now for a while,** and then you lose interest in it, and then you resume it. But actually, of course, your unconscious mind knows ahead of time when you are going to lose your interest, and it knows ahead of time when you are going to develop that interest. Actually, of course, it may seem to your conscious mind that you suddenly renewed your interest in photography because you happened to seek a particularly good photographic subject, but *if you could know what went on in your unconscious mind, you would then realize that your unconscious mind led you to take the steps in such-and-such a direction that brought you face-to-face consciously with a good photographic subject. Or, it led you to say something to somebody to elicit a response that would evoke a good photographic situation. And your conscious mind suddenly became aware of it. But your unconscious mind had slowly built it up. No matter what chance situation you find yourself in, your unconscious directs your behavior in that chance [trance?] situation, so that you suddenly see something.* And your renewal of interest in photography comes about because the unconscious enabled you to see something all of a sudden that your conscious mind could approve of for photographic purposes. And so it is in all of your behavior.

> ER: Erickson begins this section noting what may be the subject's highest level of creative intelligence and human sensibility: "At the breakfast table you mentioned the matter of portrait photographs, and the expressiveness of them, and the oversight of them." The subject in this initial stage of trance must feel deeply appreciated that the casual expression of his artistic perceptiveness at breakfast is hereby acknowledged and respected by Erickson. By the principle of ideodynamic focusing[5], any association touching upon one's highest level of sensibility tends to evoke at least some aspects of the actual experience of those levels, as well as many of the creative potentials associated with them. The subject's highest levels of potential are thereby momentarily activated; his creative possibilities are nascent and ready to react and bind with something. Erickson im-

mediately provides that "something" with the second half of the sentence, "and yet your unconscious knows when and how and why you developed that interest." The subject's activated creative impulses are now turned inward to the vast storehouse of his own unconscious—his lifetime record of experiential learnings from which will come the actual means and mechanisms of his cure.

Erickson continues this careful association of the subject's conscious interests and unconscious sources of potentials with truisms about the creative process: "No matter what chance situation you find youself in, your unconscious directs your behavior in that chance [trance?] situation so that you suddenly see something." Is Erickson making a playful and potentially therapeutic associative pun here between the words *chance* and *trance?* Or was this just a technical ambiguity in the low fidelity tape recording of his voice?

For this commentator, the subtle issues of the transference are also raised in this passage. Freud viewed the essence of transference as a more or less fortuitous mental-emotional association between current and past relationships. The patient responds to a current relationship with the analyst in a manner more appropriate to previous relationships (most typically, the parents). This overgeneralization or projection from the past helps the analyst recognize what patterns characterized the patient's past relationships, and so provides much of the material needed for "working through" the neurotic conflicts. Valid and valuable as this concept is in many situations, we must turn to C.G. Jung for a more fascinating insight into Erickson's approach of evoking the subject's highest sensibilities at this point. Jung's special contribution was the insight that the transference bond mediated the patient's "transcendent function," so that the patient clung tightly to the therapist as the only available person who recognized and reinforced his highest potentials of awareness and functioning. As Jung expressed it in his seminal paper, "The Transcendent Function"[6]:

> "The constructive or synthetic method of treatment presupposes insights which are at least potentially present in the patient... If the analyst knows nothing of these potentialities, he cannot help the patient develop them either... In actual practice, therefore, the suitably trained analyst mediates the transcendent function of the patient, i.e., helps him to bring conscious and unconscious together and so arrive at a new attitude. In this function of the analyst lies one of the many important meanings of the *transference*. The patient clings by means of the transference to the person who seems to promise him a renewal of attitude; through it he seeks this change, which is vital to him, even though he may not be conscious of doing so."

By touching upon one of the subject's highest levels of sensibility (the expressiveness of portrait photographs), Erickson is indirectly activating transference processes that are involved in the creation of new levels of awareness, as well as in the utilization of those mechanisms and processes needed for symptom cure.

Accessing the Creative Unconcious

Therapeutic Analogies of the Creative Unconscious Bypassing Conscious Learned Limitations; Reframing Perfectionism; A Concise Demonstration of the Indirect Therapeutic Approach

E: A patient comes to you and says, "I do not know what to talk about; my mind is a blank." And you point to the bookcase across the room and tell him, "Never examine the books. Just go over, reach out with your left hand if you're right-handed, and pick out the first book that your hand happens to touch. Don't try to read the title, but just pick out the first book that your hand happens to touch. And what book is selected? One patient "accidentally" picked out a book entitled, *The Startle Pattern*. What was the purpose of that? The patient had startle reactions and panic

reactions—he was forever getting startled. When did the patient read that title? I really don't know. But the patient was interested in the title consciously and asked, "What does it mean?" But his unconscious knew.

The patient tells you all about his difficulties at work, disclaiming any other problems, when he "accidentally" picks out a book entitled, *Social Problems*. Yet the patient tells you, "It's only a work problem—I have no social difficulties." Innumerable such instances could be cited. You see, *the unconscious mind knows a great deal about the problem but has difficulty in getting the conscious mind willing to let it function. The conscious mind says, "I'm a perfectionist, and I must do it this way," without recognizing that being a perfectionist enables you to do things in a great variety of ways—not just one, selected, conscious way.*

> ER: Erickson has apparently picked up a perfectionistic characteristic as a learned limitation in this subject's personality. One becomes a perfectionist as a defense against feelings of inadequacy and vulnerability. Perfectionism is a learned limitation of the conscious mind that inhibits creativity by imposing standards of the past on the flux of the ever-present new. Erickson attempts to depotentiate this learned limitation of the subject's rigid conscious mental set by giving two examples of how the unconscious went unerringly to the heart of a problem that had eluded conscious understanding. In these two therapeutic analogies, giving into the guidance of the unconscious is emphasized with: "Never examine the books [consciously]... Reach out with your *left* [the unconscious side] hand if you're right-handed."
>
> This opens an avenue for reframing the defensive learned limitation of perfectionism into its reverse: "Being a perfectionist enables you to do things in a great variety of ways—not just one, selected, conscious way." What a surprising turnabout! Erickson does not label the subject's personality characteristic of perfectionism as a problem—he does not supply an iatrogenic reinforcement by discussing it as a personal deficit. Maybe the subject never thought of

himself as perfectionistic. Why then should a doctor label, reify, and reinforce such a limiting viewpoint? Erickson avoids this trap by mentioning perfectionism as a generic characteristic of conscious thinking, and then moves quickly to reframe it in a thoroughly positive way.

This is a very concise demonstration of Erickson's indirect therapeutic approach: (1) dissociate and momentarily liberate the subject from his problem by discussing it as happening to someone else; (2) use a few therapeutic analogies to illustrate how natural unconscious processes can bypass the learned limitations that define the problem; (3) reframe the problem into a broader context that reveals the creative, healthy intent latent within it, so that (4) the problem behavior or symptom is redefined as a useful signal of an important choice point—a growing edge of some aspect of the subject's individuality and evolving competence. Thus what was a behavioral deficit becomes an asset—a cue prompting consciousness to its potentials—to its broadest possibilities of choice.

Secrets and the Inner Life

"Secrets" and the Activation of Mental Dynamics for Therapeutic Work: Covering All Possibilities of Response: Resistance and Permissive Possibilities; Indirectly Facilitating Rapport

E: Now I want you to go deeply into a trance, and very deeply. *Not necessarily "deeply" as you consciously understand it, but "deeply" as your unconscious mind can understand.* **And I think it should be interesting to you** *consciously to discover many things that your unconscious mind already knows and is willing to share with you.*

[Pause]

Consciously you can get bored, indifferent, relaxed, curious, resentful, antagonistic in any way. **And that is entertain-**

ing to you as the conscious personality. You may go into a sleep consciously, if that is interesting to you. But I think you should recognize that I want to talk primarily to your unconscious, and that I will try to talk in such a way that your unconscious understands a great deal more than your conscious mind does. *Because your unconscious mind should have many secrets from me,*

[Pause]

many secrets from you consciously, in order to get you to function more adequately.

> ER: What curious talk! But it is all true, apparently. Of course one cannot go into trance as the conscious mind understands it—the conscious mind cannot understand trance. Only the unconscious understands the mechanisms of sleep, altered states, and trance. And certainly it will be interesting for the conscious mind "to discover many things that your unconscious mind already knows and is willing to share with you." How could it be otherwise? All of these indisputable truisms continue to reinforce the *yes set* of accepting the leading role of the unconscious.
> What is the subject actually experiencing at this moment? Erickson may not be sure, but perhaps he senses some resistance so he jumps in with a suggestion that covers all possibilities of response: "consciously you can get bored, indifferent, relaxed, curious, resentful, antagonistic in any way." Enough is covered in this seemingly casual and permissive suggestion to put Erickson into positive rapport with just about anything the subject could be experiencing consciously. Erickson would never belabor a subject with the presumptuous and obnoxious direct command, "You will now be in complete rapport with me." Who wouldn't shrink from such demand! Rather Erickson suggests permissive possibilities almost any of us would be

willing to accept—without quite realizing we had thereby also indirectly accepted a positive rapport with him.

But what is the purpose of that final sentence, "Because your unconscious mind should have many *secrets* from me, [pause] many *secrets* from you consciously, in order to get you to function more adequately"? *Secrets* is a very evocative word which Erickson uses twice in the same sentence, with a careful pause in between. This cannot be an accident; something very important is being offered. On one level we can recognize a basic truism of mental functioning: the unconscious does have secrets; it does have ways and means of functioning that the conscious mind is never aware of; it does have "secrets" that would only be clutter to the conscious mind. But on another level *secrets* is a word in our society that is loaded with many evocative and energizing meanings. Whatever secret guilts and hidden anxieties the subject may have, they are now touched upon and ideodynamically activated by use of the word *secrets*. Erickson is thus building up a high energy charge that (1) continues to reinforce the *yes set* for dominance of unconscious processes, and (2) provides the mental activation and driving force for the therapeutic work that is to be done. The mental energy locked up in the subject's secrets and their defense is now being channeled along a path of therapeutic utility. There is really no passive aspect to Erickson's use of hypnosis: *therapeutic trance is a state of heightened mental activation designed to do important therapeutic work.*

Diagramming Associative Networks Initiating Therapeutic Trance

Following is a diagram of the associative networks utilized by Erickson to initiate therapeutic trance in the subject throughout Section I.

```
   ┌─────────────┐                          ┌─────────────┐
   │ CONSCIOUS   │ ───────────────────────→ │ UNCONSCIOUS │
   │ INTERESTS   │                          │ INTEREST    │
   └─────────────┘                          └─────────────┘
```

- Yes set & truisims
- Photography & highest potentials
- Reframing perfectionism with therapeutic analogy
- Depotentiating learned limitations

- Opening flower metaphor
- Unconscious does its own thinking & feeling
- Ideodynamic focusing of therapeutic potentials
- Indirect transference
- Unconscious choice

```
                    MIND WANDERING
```

```
   ┌─────────────┐                          ┌─────────────┐
   │ COMMON EVERY│ ───────────────────────→ │ TRANCE      │
   │ DAY TRANCE  │                          │ BEGINNINGS  │
   └─────────────┘                          └─────────────┘
```

- Close eyes & relax
- Ultradian rhythms
- No effort whatsoever

- "A part you do not know"
- "It knows a tremendous amount about you"
- Healing by its own natural processes

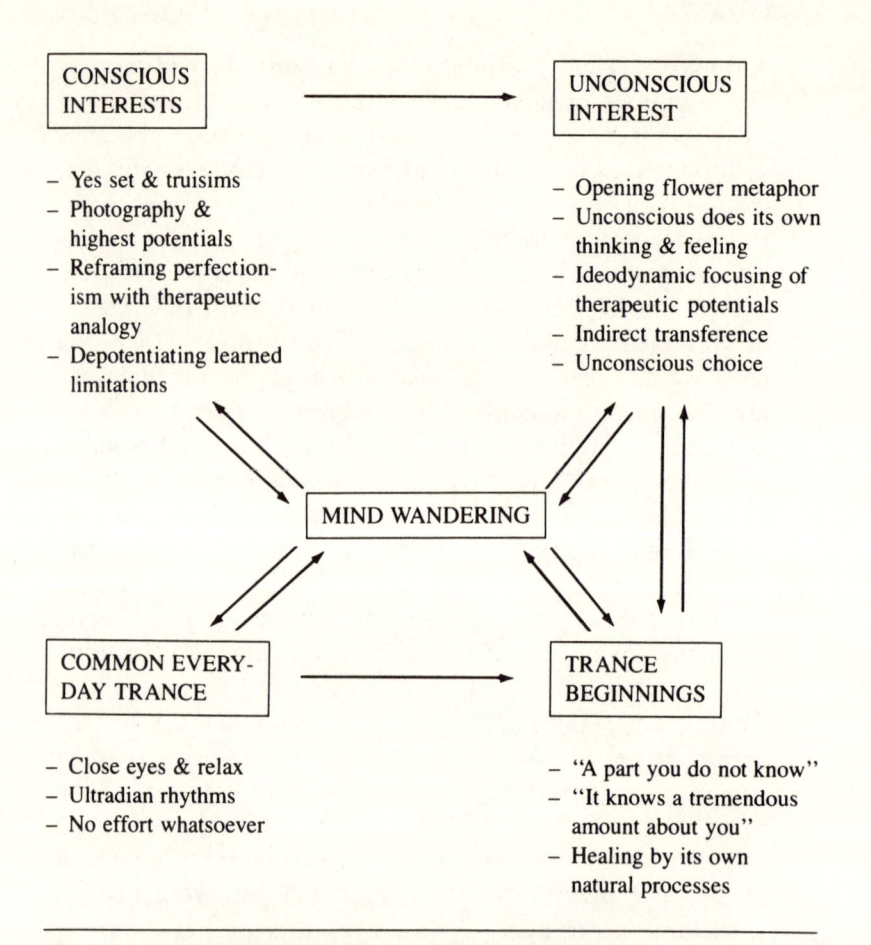

Figure 1: Only one of many possible ways to diagram some of the features involved in the *associative network initiating therapeutic trance* in Section I. All the processes enclosed in boxes are mutually supportive, with an extra shift toward Unconscious Interest and Trance Beginnings.

SECTION II

EVOKING UNCONSCIOUS POTENTIALS

Utilization Theory

Questions and Therapeutic Analogies Evoking Individuality: Reframing Disturbances into Utilities: Wondering as an Inner Search

E: **What are the things that your unconscious can do? Sometimes the stenographer can type more rapidly if she chews gum, yet chewing gum is no part of typing except for her. Some stenographers can type more rapidly in a room by themselves, and others type more rapidly in the presence of others where there is a disturbing noise. [Erickson is coughing at this point.]** *We do not judge that this or that thing is necessarily disturbing. We only wonder what use can be made of it.*

> ER: Having activated the subject's inner processes in the previous sections, Erickson is now able to pop the important question, "What are the things that your unconscious can do?" He adds the illustration of a stenographer typing more rapidly if she chews gum as a therapeutic analogy to evoke the subject's own idiosyncracies as tools and facilitating correlates of his unique styles of creativity.
>
> Erickson has a disturbing cough at this point and immediately utilizes it for the subject's potential benefit by reframing the disturbance into a possible utility. As he says so succinctly, "We do not judge that this or that thing is necessarily disturbing. We only *wonder* what use can be made of it." Within these two simple sentences is the essence of what Erickson called the *utilization theory* of psychotherapy.[7] Too often our conscious minds limit us by judging situations and stimuli as negative and worthless—

257

as things to be avoided or overcome. Erickson would rather have us *wonder* about them. The process of wondering is actually a quiet inner search for a creative response from the unconscious that can reframe and utilize the so-called disturbance.

Teaching Trance Deepening

Offering the Unconscious Possibilities of Hypnotic Exploration and Altered Sensory-Perceptual Modes of Experience; Hand Levitation; Ideas as Concrete Realities

E: *In teaching you to be willing to learn how to go more and more deeply into trance, I think that your unconscious should have the privilege of letting you develop hand levitation. Whether you know what that means or not isn't really important.* Or perhaps your unconscious might want you to discover that your hands are numb and feelingless; or perhaps it might want to bring about a numb, feelingless condition in your hands and arms while you were consciously convinced that it did not exist. You see, consciously we learn to deal with concrete reality. Consciously we can shift a table: we put our hands on it and we move it across the floor, which we can feel with our feet and hands and see with our eyes. And we can lift the table. We can sense its hardness, its weight, and we can appreciate its color—all concrete realities. But in our mind's eye we can still deal with that table, and in our mind's eye we can close our eyes and see that table. We do not need to touch it. We can sense the feeling of that table in our hands; we can sense the feeling of movement in our feet even while sitting perfectly still. *The unconscious mind deals with ideas, with memories, with understandings; and it is not important that the unconscious mind causes the body to get up and walk across the floor and pick up the table to move it, because the unconscious mind can deal with those ideas, and those ideas are as concrete as the table itself.*

ER: Erickson's words here are the clearest expression of his understanding of the trance deepening process. There is nothing magical about it; Erickson simply *teaches a willingness to learn how to let the unconscious have more privileges.* Who can argue against having more privileges? He then offers numerous hypnotic or altered modes of functioning for the subject's possible exploration. These altered modes of functioning will naturally occur once the conscious ego gives up its learned habitual activity of constructing a consensually correct or veridical concrete reality. How boring it must be for the enslaved potentials of our creative unconscious to continually serve the prosaic and mundane needs of this so-called "consensual reality"! No wonder the unconscious goes off on a binge now and then in its natural strivings for some form of original self-expression. Usually we manacle its efforts so severely in the name of "reality" that the best it can do is serve us up some sort of pathetic individual expression that we promptly label as a "neurotic symptom," or worse.[8]

The truth is that the province of the unconscious is the realm of ideas, and therein it can be as creative as it is allowed to be. Once freed from the constraints of so-called outer consensual reality, the unconscious can reorganize and reframe ideas, perceptions, feelings, and behaviors in infinite variety, and in any therapeutic fashion. After the unconscious has made these therapeutic reorganizations within itself, it is then available to support our conscious ego's need to build consensual realities that bridge our interactions with the outer world.

Dreaming as Self-Creation

Dreams as a Therapeutic Analogy of Individuality and Trance: Memory Images as the Reality of Mental Life: Consensual Reality in General Terms Only: The Picture Metaphor of Individual Experience

E: In one's dreams at night, the dream can be very vivid, very real. One can drive a car, one can talk to friends, one

can visit with people who have long been forgotten, one can re-visit the scenes of childhood in the dream. And it is a very, very real mental experience to have that dream. Because *the memory images are the realities of the mental life of any person. And in a trance state the essential thing is to deal with those concrete realities of mental experience. They need not be the tangible items of reality that everybody else can experience; they have to be those realities of individual experience. The picture that you take and show me is a picture that I see with a different pair of eyes,* with a different background, with a different understanding, and it is a different picture that I see. Only the paper is the same. And I see a different expression on that photograph; I see a different meaning, a different value as very real to me. But only I can see that. And only you can see what you see. *We can agree in certain general terms, but that is all.*

> ER: The major theme of freeing individual creativity from the constraints of a rigid reliance on outer consensual reality is continued in this section by using dreams as a therapeutic analogy: "Memory images are the realities of the mental life of any person." It is these memory images that are the real stuff of mental life and of hypnotherapeutic work. Imagination in the sense of a purely fanciful construction has a place in therapeutic work, but it is the real "memory images" that Erickson seeks to engage and work with. The reality of memory images was an original discovery made by Erickson as a 17-year-old youth paralyzed throughout his body by an acute attack of poliomyelitis. In a self-conceived rehabilitation program, Erickson used his real memory images of movement to retrain his muscles and regain full body mobility.[9]
>
> Erickson then gives expression to the philosophical truths of our relative realities in terms a photographer can certainly understand: "The picture that you take and show me is a picture that I see with a different pair of eyes... We can agree in general terms, but that is all." Consensual reality exists only in general terms. Most of us waste too

much of our creative energy trying to impose our view on others in the illusion that what *we* believe is an objective truth. This is what is called *power* in twentieth-century consciousness: seeking to construct mental realities that others must abide by. Yet as Erickson so profoundly points out, this notion of objective reality is an illusion: we cannot really be sure we are seeing the same thing when looking at a photograph through two different pairs of eyes. How much more delusionary, then, is this so-called power of enforcing a purportedly collectively determined consensual reality as a way of life for all? It can't be done; only its illusion can be perpetrated through confrontation, force, and fight. How much better to appreciate the usefulness of each of us constructing our own varieties of "reality" for our own particular purposes—purposes based on individual patterns of needs, learnings, potentials, and abilities. The resulting individual patterns of skill can then be shared to mutual and collective advantage when needed.

Altered States in Everyday Life

Utilizing "Wondering" and "Staring" for Trance Deepening;
Evoking Visual Hallucinatory Mechanisms: Real Memory
Images and Associative Networks for Activating Potentials and
Early Learning Sets: A Diagram

E: As you sit there I would like to have you go deeper and deeper into the trance; to be willing mentally to find yourself standing before a window looking out into the distance, *wondering what you will see, what you will feel.* **One can think of landscape scenes, city scenes, of flowers and trees, of cars, an expanse of water, mountains, fog—who knows? And** *it would be delightful as a personal experience to stand and stare out of the window and let come to mind whatever visual memory, visual image, that wishes.* **The unconscious mind can reach back into the past, or it can reach out into one's understanding of the future, because one's understand-**

ing of the future has to be framed in current understandings interpolated in terms of future times.

I can ask that you *see yourself lying flat on a bed in the late afternoon wondering—as you have in the past without realizing it now consciously—wondering which hand is your right hand, and which hand is your left hand. You've had that experience, whether you remember it consciously or not. Just wondering, and really wondering which hand is the right, which is the left, because that is something that really did happen to you long ago when you were trying to identify your [body parts]. And as all children do, you wondered how many feet you had while you were trying to form a concept of two, and to differentiate two from three, and one from five.* There are so many things that you take for granted as established. You must also recognize that there are a lot of other things established in your mental experience—things that may seem absurd, such as which is really your right hand, which is really your left hand. You see, the simple identification of the right hand does not mean the identification of the left hand. There was a time when both your right hand and your left hand seemed to be just two right hands, or just two left hands, or just two hands, or just one hand. And *those memory images were very real personal experiences and understandings.*

I do not know very much about you, but your unconscious knows a great deal. I can suggest motor activity to you; I can suggest walking across the floor; picking up a book and reading it; [focusing] with a camera; driving a car; waiting for a bus; wondering what you are going to eat; being unwilling to take off your shoes to go to bed. *I can suggest any number of things, but the purpose of my suggestions is to let your unconscious discover its own range of things.*

> ER: Once again we find Erickson talking about "wondering what you will see, what you will feel" as a permissive, questioning approach to trance deepening. This open-ended wondering functions as an indirect suggestion for evoking almost any personal response, which in turn

establishes further response readiness: whatever response the subject makes will be automatically associated with Erickson's suggestion and thus reinforce the tendency to respond positively to further suggestions. Erickson adds that "it would be delightful as a personal experience to stand and stare out of the window and let come to mind whatever visual memory, visual image, that wishes." Standing and staring out the window (along with wondering) are, in fact, very common altered experiences in everyday life that we have all experienced. Erickson now deepens the subject's trance by touching upon them here in the context of evoking visual memory images that could be used later in the subject's possible experience of visual hallucinations. Who has not lain "flat on a bed in the late afternoon wondering... "? Who has not fallen half asleep at such times and experienced spontaneous hypnogogic states involving dreams and distortions of body image and feeling?

But then Erickson does something radically surprising in a very casual manner: he associates these common hypnogogic experiences in the late afternoon with a child's earliest experiences of "wondering—as you have in the past without realizing it consciously—wondering which hand is your right hand, and which is your left hand... And as all children do, you wonder how many feet you have while you are trying to form the concept of two, and to differentiate two from three, and one from five." What is Erickson doing with such associations? Many things all at the same time! He is building another associative network which links many levels of experience and responsiveness together. He is building a triadic bridge of associations between (1) the current state of trance deepening, (2) the common everyday trance experience, and (3) the subject's earliest years of unconscious learnings. These earliest and most profound learning sets "trying to form a concept of two, and to differentiate two from three, and one from five," are evoked and brought up to the current trance situation, both as metaphors and as activated early learning

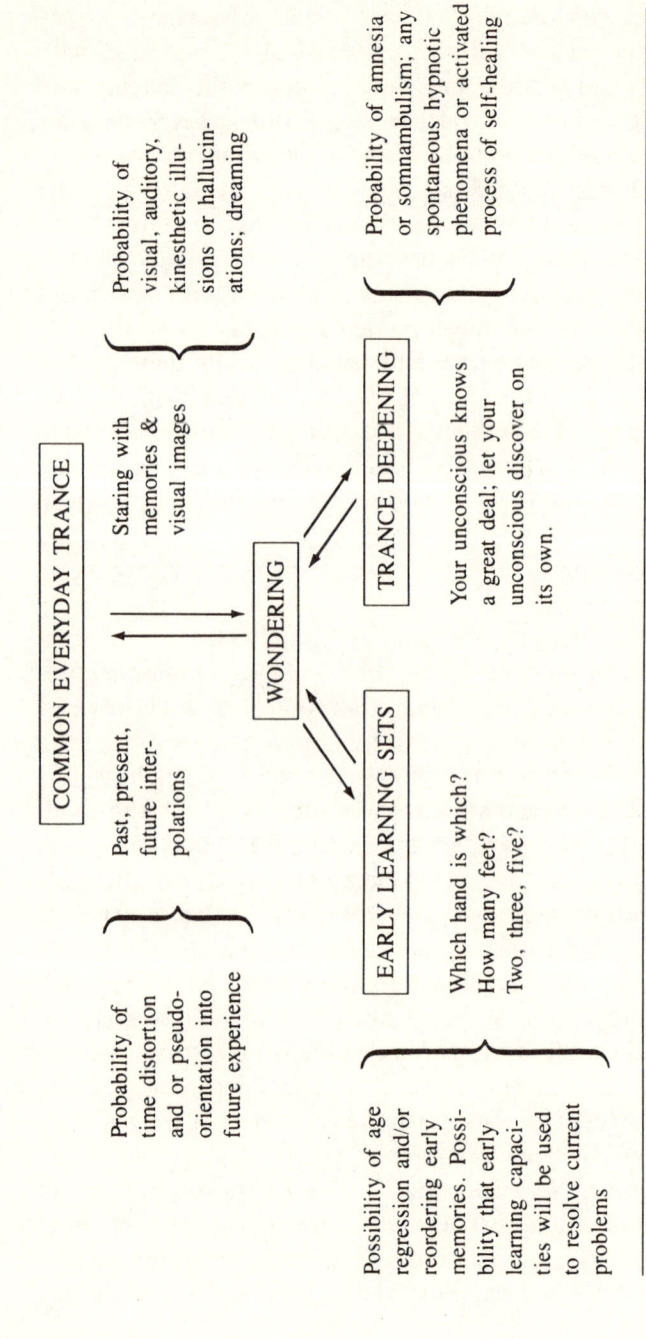

COMMON EVERYDAY TRANCE

| Probability of time distortion and or pseudo-orientation into future experience | Past, present, future interpolations | Staring with memories & visual images | Probability of visual, auditory, kinesthetic illusions or hallucinations; dreaming |

⇅

WONDERING

⇅   ⇅

EARLY LEARNING SETS	**TRANCE DEEPENING**
Which hand is which? How many feet? Two, three, five?	Your unconscious knows a great deal; let your unconscious discover on its own.

| Possibility of age regression and/or reordering early memories. Possibility that early learning capacities will be used to resolve current problems | Probability of amnesia or somnambulism; any spontaneous hypnotic phenomena or activated process of self-healing |

Figure 2: An associative network between current trance deepening, the common everyday trance, and exploratory early learning sets evident in Section II. Note how Erickson is setting up *a priori* conditions (by evoking memory images ideodynamically) that will enhance the probability of the subject experiencing any variety of hypnotic phenomena, depending on the subject's own predispositions at the moment he is receiving Erickson's suggestion. *Wondering* is the common denominator whereby each part of the associative network can evoke, facilitate, reinforce, and be supported by the other.

264

sets that may be used to explore and solve current problems.

Erickson then summarizes and reinforces this whole network of associations with the suggestion, "I can suggest any number of things, but the purpose of my suggestions is to let your unconscious discover its own range of things." This final sentence at once constellates the new associative networks as "reified" mental realities while giving the unconscious "free reign" to "discover its own range of things" from among them. An outline of the associative network that is developing is presented in Figure 2. Note how open-ended is the entire framework of Erickson's suggestions. All suggestions are designed to enhance and mutually reinforce the probability of experiencing a variety of hypnotic phenomena. So complex are the possible interactions between the therapist's suggestion and the subject's experience that the practice of hypnotherapy is best understood as *an art of enhancing probabilities* rather than as a science of deterministic and mechanistic responses. Because of this, the therapist's skill in observing and testing which suggestions the subject is beginning to respond to is of essence in the process of further extending, reinforcing, and channeling those suggestions into therapeutic avenues.

SECTION III

FACILITATING ACTIVE TRANCE WORK

Discharging Resistance

A Curiously Concise Labeling of Conscious Resistance: The Conscious/Unconscious Double Bind?

E: *Now consciously you will want to be honest and fair. You are not to deceive Dr. H or me. And consciously you will try to defend, when actually what is needed is the cooperation of your unconscious.*

> ER: This appears to be a curiously concise labeling and discharging of resistance. Of course the subject is consciously trying to be "honest and fair" and is not out "to deceive Dr. H or me." Erickson can read this in the subject's obvious behavioral efforts to be sincere. Yet human nature being what it is, we must assume that even honest subjects—especially "honest and fair" nice-guy-type-subjects—will also have typical characteriological defenses. So they will "consciously... try to defend" in thought if not in deed. This very characteristic struggle of the hypnotic subject to be honest and fair and yet defend is neatly recognized, labeled, and then summarily dismissed by Erickson when he concludes with, "... when actually what is needed is the cooperation of your unconscious."
>
> There appears to be a conscious/unconscious double bind in Erickson's labeling of the conscious conflict:

"*Consciously* you will want to be honest and fair. You are not to deceive Dr. H or me."	Vs.	"*Consciously* you will try to defend."

Both of these conflicts are made irrelevant and thereby depotentiated by what is really important for the subject.

"... when actually what is needed is the cooperation of your *unconscious.*"

This could be seen as a double bind because no matter which side of the *conscious* conflict the subject is experiencing, it tends to be depotentiated by the overwhelmingly greater significance of the needed cooperation of the *unconscious.* If the subject implicitly accepts without question the need for his unconscious cooperation, than his conscious conflict with its potential resistance is rendered irrelevant and therefore no longer in control of his experience and behavior.

We can now understand why Erickson spent so much effort in many of the previous sections building the wide-ranging associative network (see Figures 1 and 2) that strongly bound and reinforced the subject's belief in the need for his own unconscious cooperation. In Bateson's terminology, the subject's belief in the need for activation of his own unconscious (which holds the key to his healing) now functions as a *metalevel* in controlling and depotentiating any conflict or resistance on the conscious *object level* of whatever the subject happens to be thinking about the matter. We will see in the next section how Erickson continues to build and reinforce this belief in the therapeutically controlling aspect of the unconscious via the presentation of yet another therapeutic analogy.

Margaret Ryan (MR): I'm still not convinced that this is a conscious-unconscious double bind. For me the unconscious part ("when actually what is needed is the cooperation of your unconscious") would have to be an inevitability rather than a contingency to make this a bind. As it stands, the depotentiation of the subject's conscious conflict rests only on a contingency of his prior acceptance of the need for unconscious cooperation. I thought the conscious part would have to inevitably imply the unconscious part in order for this to be a bind.

ER: Ryan's lack of conviction here is entirely appropriate and illustrates the central difficulties in the practical clinical use of the double bind. A double bind exists only if the subject already has the critical metalevel (in this case, the controlling belief in the needed therapeutic cooperation of the unconscious) operating within. It was my judgment that Erickson had already built it in. It is an equally valid judgment, however, to argue that Erickson is still in the process of building it in. At this point we really have no way to determine which judgment is correct.

This uncertainty about whether or not the critical metalevel that does the binding is present and currently active within the subject is what makes the clinical use of the double bind such a chancy proposition. Bateson (in a personal communication) has compared the double bind to the joke. People really laugh at a joke only if the punch line suddenly topples an already built-in and fully accepted world view. A double bind binds only if the subject has a certain "punch line"—a critical metalevel already operating within that accepts and completes the alternatives that the therapist is offering for its double binding possibilities.[10]

Trance Without Awareness

The Ultradian Hypothesis and the Common Everyday Trance; Active Trance Work Versus Passive Cooperation: an Indirect Suggestion for Unconscious Work

E: *A patient who tells me most emphatically that he has not been in a trance, and really believes it,* **and can prove it in a half dozen ways, convincingly,** *may nevertheless have been in a deep trance and is keeping that knowledge very carefully from me and from the self, so that the unconscious could better use the experience for its own purposes. And it isn't a question of being honest or sincere or cooperating. It is* *merely a matter of the unconscious doing things in the way that is best for it.*

> ER: Very subtle phenomenological issues are raised in this section. Most of us simply do not recognize our altered states—the common everyday trance experiences—in the normal flow of daily activity. In fact, however, our consciousness is constantly shifting in its focus between attention to outer and inner worlds. In spite of this most of us experience the illusion that our consciousness is one unbroken and seamless whole—with no gaps of altered states in it. We have the illusion that we (our conscious ego intentionality) control this consciousness and can shift it about at will, even turning it off and on when we sleep and awake. In actual fact the minimal command we have over the contents of our consciousness is probably just enough to foster the illusion of more total control. Erickson apparently believes that the purpose (survival value) of this illusion is "that the unconscious could better use the experience [of creative trance] for its own purposes.
>
> Our ultradian hypothesis helps us understand that the common everyday trance is part of a natural oscillation in the focus of consciousness between the outer and the inner.[11] When we fall into the inner-focus phase every 90 minutes or so, we are probably under the sway of parasympathetic and right-hemispheric processes. These processes do a great deal of the internal "bookkeeping" (outside the normal range of consciousness, of course) that ultimately supports our periods of outer focus as well. For the purposes of therapeutic trance, I believe it is typically the inner-focus phase of the ultradian cycle that Erickson is interested in to gain access to the individual's repository of life experience in order to facilitate that "reassociation and reorganization of ideas, understandings, and memories so essential for an actual cure."[12]
>
> Erickson is thus giving clear expression to his theory of healing when he continues with: "And it isn't a question of

being honest or sincere or cooperating. It is merely a matter of the unconscious doing things in the way that is best for it." Many cooperative subjects believe that just being cooperative is enough. Hypnotherapists also fall into the same error and wonder why their cooperative, apparently "deep trance" patients do not improve. Passive complaisance is not enough! Erickson spent much effort learning to distinguish between passive responsiveness or complaisance—wherein the subject was merely cooperating—and the more genuine manifestations of an active trance state—wherein more genuine hypnotic phenomena were experienced autonomously. Of course, it is in the active trance states that the more profound therapeutic work is accomplished.[13] In this section Erickson recognizes that the subject may be merely cooperating, and Erickson probably feels he must compensate by emphasizing that the unconscious needs to do—*work!* That is the hidden implication—the really important indirect suggestion—which is interspersed between-the-lines in this seemingly gentle series of truisms about the unconscious.

Childhood as a Therapeutic Metaphor

Activating Metalevels of Motivation to Energize the Therapeutic Process: Obstinacy Reframed as "Wanting to Want"

E: There is the child who insists that he must have a toy to go to bed with, and rejects every toy in the house. Mother gets disgusted and Daddy gets disgusted, and yet if they really wanted to recognize the situation, *the child didn't really want a toy. The child merely wanted to want a toy.* **And the child could only want to want a toy by stating that he wanted a toy, and then rejecting every one. But the child was seeking the experience of** *wanting to want.* **And the parent who understands this promptly meets the situation by letting the child want to want.**

ER: Even more subtle phenomenological issues are raised in this passage. Erickson offers a typical homily of home-life—a child wanting to want a toy—as a possible way of activating early childhood metalevels of motivation. Metalevels of motivation?! Whoever heard of such a thing? Would Erickson turn over in his grave if he could see how we are carrying on, labeling his humble, homespun tales with yet another level of phenomenological esoterica?

But does not "wanting to want" describe a metalevel of wanting? I am sure Erickson never thought of it as such. He never used such concepts in his writings and teaching, and indeed, he did not seem particularly concerned about them. Yet his actual work implies an intuitive understanding of the role of metalevels in human behavior. The concept of metalevels had been used in the foundations of modern mathematics[14] half a century earlier, but no one had used it in psychology. No one, that is, except for Gregory Bateson who adopted *metalevels* as a way of conceptualizing the disturbed communication processes in schizophrenia. No wonder Bateson and his colleagues found an early ally in Erickson, who had been using metalevels and double binds constructively all of his life—even though he did not label them as such.

What is the purpose of activating early childhood metalevels of motivation? Erickson is apparently trying to evoke an emotional charge; he is evoking the energy source of life's earliest strivings in order to utilize them to fuel the subject's current therapeutic process.

MR: I had another impression of the meaning of this passage. In addition to activating metalevels of motivation, Erickson seems to be reframing childhood behavior normally judged to be obstinate, intractable, or self-centered as serving the positive function of experiencing a "wanting to want." There seems to be a subtle tie-in here with his earlier reframing of perfectionism [Section I]. In both cases he is attempting to reframe and rechannel the energy bound in negative and self-defeating expressions of motivation into the therapeutic process.

The Difference Between Therapeutic and Stage Hypnosis

Freedom to Do Unconscious Work Versus Ego-Enhancing Needs of the Stage Hypnotist

E: No matter what you think consciously, the important thing is what your unconscious thinks and how it does that thinking. And whether you know it or not, you are sleeping deeply enough for your unconscious to achieve a great variety of things. And what are those things? *They are not necessarily that of giving a stage demonstration of hypnosis—that is not the purpose of this morning's work. The purpose of this morning's work is to let your unconscious have a feeling of freedom, a feeling that it wants to do things, perhaps with your knowledge and perhaps without your knowledge.*

ER: Here Erickson touches upon a fundamental issue in hypnosis: the subject's purpose is "not necessarily that of giving a demonstration of stage hypnosis," but rather to experience his unconscious freedom to do things without the limitations of his conscious knowledge. The fundamental antithesis between stage hypnosis and therapeutic hypnosis is that in therapeutic work the patient's unconscious is freed to do its own work for its own purposes, while in stage hypnosis the unconscious is used for the purposes of the stage hypnotist. In therapeutic work power is given to the patient's unconscious; in stage hypnosis power is all too often used to serve the ego of the stage hypnotist. The role of the stage hypnotist is particularly egregious because it only reinforces the pathology of alienating unconscious processes from their naturally therapeutic channels. Actual harmful effects can result from the demonstrations of stage hypnosis. For example, Erickson reported on "Stage Hypnotist Back Syndrome,"[15] wherein subjects who had submitted to the popular stage demonstration of suspending their cataleptic bodies in a bridge-like fashion between two chairs later sought medical aid for lower back pain.

Posthypnotic Suggestion

Suggesting "Unexpected Things" as an Implication for Therapeutic Work; Providing "Rational Reason" to Support Hypnotic Source Amnesias

E: But you are sleeping sufficiently deeply now so that *after awakening you can do a number of unexpected things, and you can do them for utterly rational reasons.* For example, after you have awakened you could actually get up, pick up my box of cigarettes, and state that you are curious about the box and the number of cigarettes that must have been in it—and all the time think that your questions were just a matter of intellectual curiosity. And you could prove it with your statements that you wanted to know the brand, the number of cigarettes in it, and really believe. While at the same time your unconscious could achieve the purpose of closing the box and putting it definitely out of my reach, or accidentally dropping it and spilling the cigarettes, or putting it in Dr. H's reach, or actually doing anything other than satisfying intellectual curiosity.

ER: One of Erickson's major contributions to the facilitation of posthypnotic suggestion was his emphasis on associating them with behavioral inevitabilities.[16] It is inevitable that a subject will later eat and sleep, wake up, go to the bathroom, etc. If the therapist associates posthypnotic suggestions with such inevitable behavioral patterns, these behaviors can serve as cues to reinforce the posthypnotic suggestion.

In this section Erickson is demonstrating another support system for posthypnotic suggestion: that of "rational reasons." It is not only inevitable that most subjects will later be involved with rational reasons, but rationality can also act as a cloak and defense which allows a subject to carry out posthypnotic suggestions with the full support of the conscious mind. By providing this rational support for carrying out the posthypnotic suggestion, the subject tends to experience a source amnesia for the origin of the suggestion. Thus the possibility of hypnotic amnesia is also reinforced.[17]

MR: Erickson may be linking "unexpected things" (unconscious work) with "rational reasons" (conscious thinking) to set up a pattern in the patient for allowing *unexpected solutions* to break through without interference from conscious (rational) judgment. This is his basic model for hypnotherapeutic work. Here he uses what is a behavioral inevitability for the subject (cigarette smoking) as the overt or behavioral correlate for the more important implicit activity of unconscious work in the problem area. If the subject follows through on the posthypnotic suggestion regarding the cigarettes, the implication may be that he is allowing similar processes to work in therapeutic areas. Carrying out the posthypnotic behavior then functions as a cue that the deeper implications for therapeutic work have been comprehended and accepted on an unconscious level. In the next section Erickson continues to provide another posthypnotic suggestion to model even more clearly the therapeutic need for the unconscious to intrude with its own autonomous activity.

Rehearsing via Posthypnotic Suggestion

Providing Analogical Behavioral Excercises in the Introjection of Autonomous Unconscious Activity: Multilevel Suggestions

E: **You are sleeping sufficiently deeply now so that if Dr. H were to snap his fingers,** *you could suddenly think that it was nighttime.* **You could go and turn on the light,** **and swear that you did not do it, because the turning on of the light would be a part of the thought,** *This is nighttime,* **and it would not be a part of your general conscious understanding that this is daytime.** *It would simply be an introjected form of activity.*

ER & MR: What is the purpose of this curious posthypnotic suggestion for the subject to suddenly think that it is nighttime and turn on the light? When Erickson follows this up with the statement, "It would simply be an introjected form of activity," it really appears to confirm Ryan's view that he is using posthypnotic suggestion as a therapeutic behavioral exercise for rehearsing the introjection of spontaneous autonomous unconscious activity.

Erickson was very fond of using simple practice and rehearsal to teach patients how to learn on many levels. He often gave the example of training a new horse to plow by hitching it between already well-trained horses. In his hypnotic demonstrations he frequently placed a first-time hypnotic subject in a chair between two well-experienced subjects. To facilitate a *yes set* for trance deepening, he would sometimes give patients a whole series of questions to which they could easily answer yes so that they would almost automatically respond with a yes to his request for them to go into trance.

In this and the previous section he is giving posthypnotic suggestions to rehearse the possibility of the unconscious intruding spontaneously with its own therapeutic mechanisms. In this case he actually tells the subject that it is "an introjected form of activity." Usually he simply offered posthypnotic suggestions that functioned as forms of rehearsal for therapeutic work without the patient ever realizing it. This may account for the inexplicable quality of some of Erickson's work when both subjects and observers did not understand the implications and hidden rehearsals in Erickson's suggestions.

The effectiveness of Erickson's therapeutic work, from this point of view, depends upon his operating on two or more levels at one time.[18] Although he believed hypnosis was a special state, he did not believe that hypersuggestibility was the most important characteristic of it for the therapist.[19] Rather it was the subject's capacity to respond and operate on many levels in this special state that was important. In his daily practice, Erickson depended on activating and utilizing the patient's unconscious processes with multi-level suggestions for successful therapeutic work; he did not depend upon the so-called hypersuggestibility of the trance state.

Minimal Behavioral Cues as Therapeutic Guides

Pupillary Dilation as a Sign of Conscious Interest and Unconscious Involvement: Developing Acute Observational Abilities

E: At the table this morning you mentioned your question about the period of relaxation. Was that a conscious inquiry? You thought it was. Obviously in listening to you it was not just your conscious mind inquiring. It was your unconscious mind that brought up that subject and forced you to raise the question. There was no way for you to see your face; there was no way for you to recognize your eyes; *there was no way for you to appreciate the fact that as you mentioned that topic and discussed it slightly in different aspects, the pupils of your eyes dilated—not in accord with the lighting situation there, but in direct relationship to certain ideas that you expressed. [There was no way for you to appreciate] that your pupils dilated, that your eye muscles slowed in their behavior, that your unconscious was arresting a great deal of your behavior so that it could listen while you consciously thought only your conscious mind was in attendance.*

ER: Erickson's remarkable observations about the relation between pupillary dilation and psychological interest in this section have been independently validated by researchers who knew nothing of Erickson's previous work.[20] The pupils tend to dilate when an idea of great interest or fascination is touched upon. Often when this interest is on a more unconscious level Erickson could determine that a particular idea or issue was of greater importance than the subject's conscious mind realized. As these issues of greater unconscious interest are touched upon, the subject tends to fall into a momentary state of fixed concentration or mild cataleptic suspension—the common everyday trance—such that "your pupils dilated, your eye muscles slowed in their behavior, and your unconscious was arresting a great deal of your behavior so that it could listen while you consciously thought only your conscious mind was in attendance."

It is this type of acute behavioral observations that guided much of Erickson's therapeutic work. When he was engaged in apparently random and neutral conversation with patients, trading memories and stories about home, work, and so forth, he was actually surveying a variety of important areas of life in order to observe when the patient's pupillary, facial, and body behaviors betrayed signs of a deeper unconscious involvement. Erickson used this sensory-perceptual guidance to quickly focus on the significant issues for each individual patient. He was so proficient at this, in fact, that he often seemed to be a "wizard" at his work. Yet he always insisted that he had no particular magic or power; that he was simply an acute observer who was constantly monitoring the minimal behavioral cues that were manifestations of problematic processes in the patient.

Utilizing Natural Behavior Cues in Therapy

Posthypnotic Suggestion Utilizing Natural Pupillary Dilation; The Indirect Teaching of a Colleague; Fail-Safe Posthypnotic Suggestions Facilitating Unconscious Responsiveness

E: *In future work with you, your unconscious is going to resort to that pupillary dilation many times to let Dr. H know that your unconscious is really talking, is really listening; so that he, in watching your pupils, will recognize that he is talking to both your conscious mind and your unconscious mind; [so that he will know] that your unconscious mind has thereby invited him to say something. Now whether or not he says the right thing is not important. The mere fact that he says something, because your unconscious invited him to, and that tells your unconscious that he is being responsive, and therefore it can be responsive, too.*

> ER: Erickson is managing to do several things at once here. He is, of course, giving a series of posthypnotic suggestions about how the subject's natural pupillary behavior can be used in the future, both by his own unconscious and by his therapist, Dr. H. Erickson is thereby also teaching Dr. H an important lesson about utilizing naturalistic behavioral cues to guide his therapeutic work.
>
> It is characteristic of Erickson to utilize naturalistic patterns of behavior in his posthypnotic suggestions. As previously mentioned it was these inevitable, naturalistic patterns of behavior—and not the purported "power" or "hypersuggestibility" of the hypnotic state—that Erickson depended upon for the carrying out of hypnotherapeutic suggestion. This important and fundamental differentiation seems to be lost again and again by over-eager but naive workers who attempt to quickly emulate Erickson's effectiveness without undergoing the necessary rigors of training in the careful observation of human behavior.
>
> The subtle, fail-safe posthypnotic suggestion concerning Dr. H's future therapeutic work with the subject also deserves special notice: "Now whether or not he says the right thing is not important... because your unconscious invited him to, and that tells your unconscious that he is being responsive, and therefore it can be responsive, too." *No special or magical power in the hypnotherapist's suggestions!* Just humble efforts at suggestion that the patient's unconscious has requested and can respond to. At a basic level this is all that is required of the hypnotherapist: a sincere, therapeutic dialogue wherein the patient's unconscious is given the freedom to respond and, if necessary, to correct and even guide the therapist, who is able to recognize the voice of the unconscious via its minimal cues.

Utilization Theory

The Unconscious Conversion of Problem Energy into Constructive Use for the Total Personality: Symptoms as Important Signals

E: You want your problem corrected. And how? Certainly not by the way that you would map out consciously. Because if it could be corrected that way, you would not have your problem. *The only way you'll want it corrected is the way your unconscious wants it corrected. And that is in such a fashion that all the energy now directed into your problem can be conserved and utilized in a way that is pleasing to you as a total personality.*

> ER: This is a clear statement of utilization theory: mental energy that is bound up in symptom formation is to be rechanneled "and utilized in a way that is pleasing to you as a total personality." The word *total* is the sleeper in this suggestion. The implication of *total personality* is that it includes the unconscious, which has needs and patterns of being which the conscious mind often knows little about. Symptoms and problems are signals from the unconscious that all is not well in the "total personality." Thus symptoms are really our best friends, letting us know that we need to tune into the "total personality" for important insights into our total life situations.

Allowing the Unconscious to Do Its Own Work

Long Pauses at the Climax of Hypnotherapeutic Activation

E: Now I have been talking at length. *I do not need to talk constantly because your unconscious has heard and understood so many more things than you have, that it can very easily cease to listen to me and do its own thinking.*

[Long pause]

ER: This section ends with a *long pause:* Erickson has set in motion a heightened state of mental activation and now *pauses* to let it pursue its therapeutic course and "do its own thinking." The inner mental events of healing and transformation are presumed to be taking place during this "pregnant" pause. This long pause is thus the *climax* of the entire induction, with all of the mental activations he has facilitated up to this point.

How different this is from the old conventional view of hypnosis as a sleepily receptive state wherein the subject's mind is a blank slate, being passively impressed with the authoritative suggestions of the operator. For Erickson the most ideal hypnotherapeutic state was one of heightened activation in which the patient worked with his own mental repertory—rather than passively responding to the domineering direct suggestions of a hypnotist. One of Erickson's earliest and clearest expressions of this radically different view of the hypnotherapeutic process was presented in his 1948 paper on "Hypnotic Psychotherapy"[21]:

> Direct suggestion is based primarily, if unwittingly, upon the assumption that whatever develops in hypnosis derives from the suggestions given. It implies that the therapist has the miraculous power of effecting therapeutic changes in the patient, and disregards the fact that therapy results from an inner resynthesis of the patient's behavior achieved by the patient himself. It is true that direct suggestion can effect an alteration in the patient's behavior and result in a symptomatic cure, at least temporarily. However, such a "cure" is simply a response to the suggestion and does not entail that *reassociation and reorganization of ideas, understandings, and memories so essential for an actual cure. It is this experience of reassociating and reorganizing his own experiential life that eventuates in a cure, not the manifestation of responsive behavior which can, at best, satisfy only the observer.* (p. 38) [Italics added]

The Role of Indirect Suggestion

A Therapeutic Analogy of Color Evoking a Full Repertory of Mental Resources: Engaging Both sides of the Brain: Translating Analogy Into Rational Terms: Evoking Active Inner Work

E: *An artist patient of mine knows very definitely that he is going to paint a picture. And he enjoys getting out the pigments—the reds, and the blues, and the browns, and the golds, and the yellows, and the pinks, and the oranges. And he really enjoys doing that. Yet he is utterly pleased after he has already arranged his things to make a black and white painting.*

What part did those things play in it? No reds, no yellows, no blues, no greens—just black and white. And yet without those colors he could not have painted the black and white painting. And so he puts out those things, earnestly believing that he is going to paint a landscape of trees and flowers. But it turns out to be a rail fence crossing a snowy field, with a lone tree in the field. Why did he bring out the pigments? *In order to get the background of what that landscape was previous to the wintertime. And against that background of mental images he gets the contrast* of the snow on the field, the leafless tree, the tree without green leaves, the rail fence without the bright-colored flowers. He really sees the rail fence then, but he got out the pigments so that *he could have a comprehensive view* of the field, the rail fence, the flowers, the green leaves. And then out of it he selects the black and the white. And he can tell you honestly as he arranges the pigments: "I am going to paint a lovely landscape, a beautiful, springtime landscape." He can really believe it, and be utterly delighted with a very lovely winter landscape, and as pleased as you are.

It is what the unconscious can do. And the first time my artist friend did that, he was curious to know why he had picked out all those [pigments], but *his unconscious knew that to get a lovely picture he had better have all the mental images, all the visual memories, out of which to select. And thus he had everything available.* **He had the flowers available in the paints, to cast aside.**

[Long pause]

ER: The analogy of getting all the colors of the palette ready, even though only black and white will be used, is clearly intended to help the subject make all his inner resources available ("all the mental images, all the visual memories out of which to select") to provide a full background of support for the really important black-and-white issues to be dealt with.

It is interesting to note here that Erickson will frequently translate a complex and crucial analogy into rational terms, even while the subject is in trance. The metaphor acts as a kind of mythopoetic expression intended for right-hemispheric receptivity, but Erickson also gives the same instructions in rational terms to the left hemisphere to ensure that both "sides" of the mind are together on the work to be accomplished.

ER & MR: In this case Erickson first presents the analogy ("An artist patient of mine knows very definitely that he is going to paint a picture ... Yet he is utterly pleased after he has already arranged his things to make a black-and-white painting"), and then he proceeds to explain it—but only in part. In the paragraph that follows Erickson elaborates on the analogy and the *dynamics of painting* a winter landscape by first visualizing its history (thus hinting that the patient's own personal history needs to be brought in to solve his problem) of a springtime of colors against which the black-and-white winter comes. He then ends the section by taking the explanation one step further into the *dynamics of unconscious processes,* which contains the really important message for the subject: " ... but his unconscious knew that to get a lovely picture he had better have all the mental images, all the visual memories, out of which to select. And thus he had everything available."

Yet notice that while providing the rational mind with sufficient understanding to engage the analogical process, Erickson stops enticingly short of a full translation. He structures the situation so that the subject must take the important step of exploring the particulars of how the analogy applies to his situation. This is the step of active inner work that is of essence in hypnotherapy where the subject is to be engaged in the "reassociation and reorganization of ideas, understandings, and memories so essential for an actual cure" (see below).

ER: It is just such aspects of Erickson's approach that help us understand his intent in using the indirect forms of suggestion. The indirect forms of suggestion are not a sneaky way of manipulating the subject's mind against his conscious will. If that were the case, why did Erickson so often translate for the subject the purpose of the indirect approach he had used a few minutes, hours, days, weeks, or even months ago?[22] Rather, "the indirect forms of suggestion are facilitators of mental associations and unconscious processes"[23] which Erickson developed in his search for increasingly effective hypnotherapeutic intervention:

> The invention and systematic use of a variety of these hypnotic forms for the study and utilization of a patient's own associative structure and mental skills in ways that are outside his usual range of conscious ego control to effect therapeutic goals does appear to be one of Erickson's original contributions to the theory and practice of "suggestion."[24]

Much careful discrimination is required of the hypnotherapist, however, in order to determine the *when* and *how* of imparting such information: *when* is the patient's conscious mind ready to hear about just *how* the indirect suggestions were used to facilitate his own unconscious processes toward rechanneling the energy tied up in his symptoms into patterns more desirable for the "total personality."

Relaxation and Learning

Relaxation to Consolidate and "Set" Hypnotherapeutic Learning: The Metaphor of a Newly Built Concrete Road: Moot Questions as Facilitators of Wondering

E: **The one thing that you need to learn, and to learn very comfortably, is how pleasant it is to relax.** *And is it relaxation, or is it a kind of learning... a form of consolidation of one's gains?* **The student who studies hard finishes his lesson, puts the book aside, and leans back comfortably in his chair, stretching, relaxing, and thinking about nothing of any importance. A concrete road is built with concrete hardness. But even though it has hardened, the traffic doesn't go over it. The builder says: "You let it set. We'll let it set; it is hard now; it is hard enough to bear traffic. But you let it set and it will withstand the winter weather; it will withstand the heavy traffic much better. It is as hard now as it will ever get, but it will set." What a vague term—just what does it mean?**

> ER: The heightened state of hypnotherapeutic activation that reached its climax in the last two sections is now followed, sensibly enough, by a period of relaxation as "a form of consolidation of one's gains." New learning is "set" during periods of apparent rest in which neuro-hormonal influences interact with brain systems to modulate memory storage.[25]
>
> Erickson uses the metaphor of concrete setting with a hardness so that "it is hard enough to bear traffic... it will withstand the winter weather." The new hypnotherapeutic learning may have to withstand the stress of future experience that will seem to contradict it in the wintery seasons of one's discontent.
>
> Erickson ends this section with the musing, "What a vague term—just what does it mean?" Indeed what is he questioning here? Is he referring to the vague meaning of

the word *set?* Is he offering a moot question that may help the subject wonder and further consolidate the "reassociating and reorganizing of his own experiential life that eventuates in a cure"? Or is Erickson using the question to shift to the subject of memories in the next section?

Facilitating Mental Climax

The Autonomy of the "Lightning-Speed Mental Life" of the Unconscious: Time Distortion, Amnesia, and "Floods of Memories"

E: *We have an idea that we must think many things.* **But we should consider the speed of nerve impulses, because nerve impulses travel approximately 130,000 miles per second. Muscle movement is much slower, but thought is placed at essentially the speed of electricity. Therefore how long does it take [to think] a whole series of thought?**

You can take a pleasant trip and not think about it again for many, many years. And then suddenly someone says a single word and instantly there flashes through your mind a whole array of memories in the instant in which you recognize that the single word was spoken.

[Pause]

The mere mention of the word *limerick* to me immediately brings to my mind a doctor's thesis written on the subject, and the long, extended correspondence I had with him on the subject of his thesis, and on the subject of his anthropological studies. In the years that followed the writing of that thesis, certainly whenever I go to New York, as soon as I enter the hotel where I am going to stay—as soon as I enter a certain room there—[I know] there is going to come a terrific rush, *a flood of memories;* and I do not know what they are. *A flood of memories.* I am going to recall names

285

that I have forgotten. I am going to recall instances that I have forgotten. And I will recall them as soon as I enter that room, and I've got only a vague idea of what that room is like. It seems to me it is on the left-hand side of the corridor, and there is a table there—but I'm not at all certain. But when I do enter that room, there will be a terrific flood of memories.

So it is in the unconscious we can become aware of only a very, very, very small part of that lightning-speed mental life that we have. There will be such a rush and flood of memories, and I'll have to give time—time as measured by a watch to follow out all of the associations that go with this name and then with that name. Just as one can enter a room filled with people, and as the door opens you see everybody. And you just know that they are all people you know. But then you have to go through the laborious process of shifting your gaze from one person to the next, and attaching a name, and attaching memories.

[Long pause]

> ER: Erickson is apparently still supporting the climax of therapeutic mental activity by freeing the subject of a common misconception: "We have an idea that we must think many things..."—that we must take a lot of conscious time to review memories and do significant inner work. That is the way consciously driven associative processes are usually experienced. Actually it is true that "in the unconscious we can become aware of only a very, very, very small part of that lightning-speed mental life." Since unconscious processes can occur so rapidly, *Erickson is indirectly facilitating a possible experience of time distortion;* and since this great speed requires autonomous unconscious processes, *the subject will probably have an amnesia for much of it*—even though, paradoxically, he may be aware of the experience of a "flood of memories." The experience of a flood of memories is highly characteristic of those breakthroughs and climaxes of mental life

where important developmental shifts take place. For Freud the release of early memories was the *sine qua non* of breaking through significant mental blocks, and this apparently spontaneous release of memories is still regarded as a significant step in most forms of psychotherapy.[25]

Diagramming Active Trance Work

Following is one possible diagram of the psychodynamic factors activated by Erickson during this section of therapeutic work.

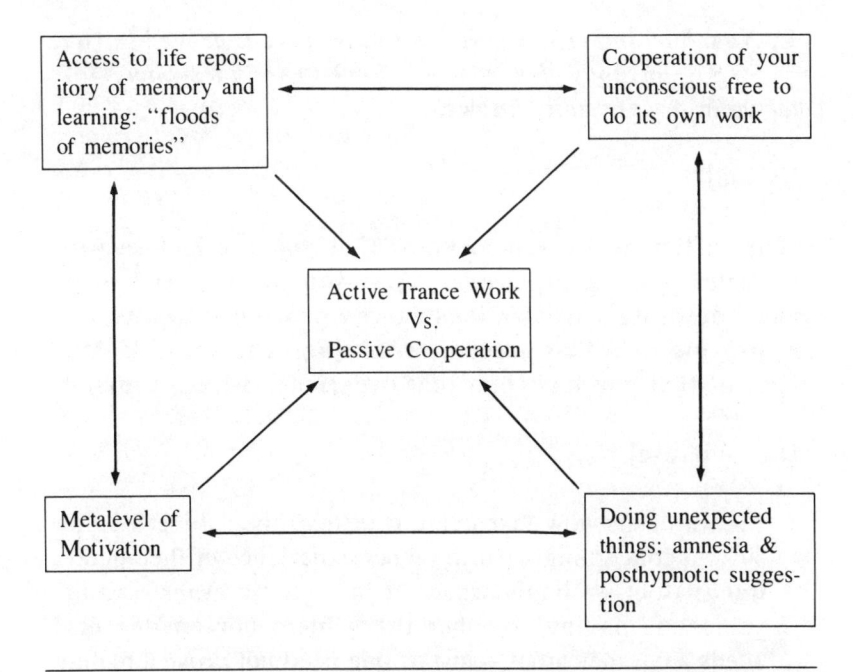

```
┌─────────────────────┐                    ┌─────────────────────┐
│ Access to life repos-│                    │ Cooperation of your │
│ itory of memory and │ ←──────────────→   │ unconscious free to │
│ learning: "floods   │                    │ do its own work     │
│ of memories"        │                    │                     │
└─────────────────────┘                    └─────────────────────┘
           ↑↓              ↘       ↙              ↑↓
                     ┌─────────────────┐
                     │ Active Trance Work│
                     │       Vs.        │
                     │ Passive Cooperation│
                     └─────────────────┘
           ↑↓              ↗       ↖              ↑↓
┌─────────────────────┐                    ┌─────────────────────┐
│ Metalevel of        │ ←──────────────→   │ Doing unexpected    │
│ Motivation          │                    │ things; amnesia &   │
│                     │                    │ posthypnotic sugges-│
│                     │                    │ tion                │
└─────────────────────┘                    └─────────────────────┘
```

Figure 3: Active trance work in Section III : An associative network of motivation, early learning sets, an unconscious "free to do its own work", and exercises to encourage its unexpected autonomous activity for that "reassociation and reorganization of ideas, understandings, and memories so essential for an actual cure."

SECTION IV

REFRAMING, POSTHYPNOTIC SUGGESTION, AND TRANCE RATIFICATION

Ratifying Trance

Experiential Metaphor of Trance as a "Prima Facie"
Therapeutic Experience

E: *Now how important is it for you to have it proved to you, or proved to anybody else, that you have been in a trance? It is what your unconscious knows.*

[Pause]

It is sufficient for you to know that you are in love with your wife. *It is an experience.* And you do not need to go around devoting a tremendous energy proving it to this person, proving it to that person, or proving it to yourself. It is sufficient that you have had that experience within yourself.

[Long pause]

> ER: Erickson now takes care to extend the subject's belief system concerning what the inner experience of therapeutic trance is: it is simply whatever therapeutic *experience* the subject is having! Neither the subject nor anyone else needs any other proof—just as one need not *prove* a feeling of love, but only *experience* it. Here Erickson is establishing inner experience as the *prima facie* of therapeutic trance. Too often people believe that an outer, behavioral (and bizarre) sensory-perceptual alteration is required in order to "prove" they have experienced trance. This is our unfortunate heritage from stage hypnosis. While it can be

entirely valid for the hypnotherapist to ratify or "prove" the existence of an altered state to the patient's conscious mind via these outer behavioral manifestations, still the best proof—and the most valuable proof—is the actual *inner experience* of the needed therapeutic effects.[26]

Facilitating Hypnotic Amnesia

Naturalistic Metaphor of Forgetting as a "Prima Facie"
Correlate of Body Processes: Forgetting Therapeutic Trance

E: *You have enjoyed eating a good dinner, enjoyed it thoroughly; and then you can forget all about having eaten a good dinner.* **It is not important that you remember eating that good dinner, nor do you need to take blood samples to prove that you are digesting the dinner. You've had the experience of eating it; you can then forget it. There's no reason why you should prove to yourself, or anybody else, that you have eaten it.** *You've had the experience; you can forget it. You can let the processes of digestion take place, but you do not need to prove that the fat is being digested; that the protein and the carbohydrates [are being digested]. There is no need even for you to remember that you've been in a trance; or even to believe that you've been in a trance.*

ER: There is an overall consistency we can discern here as we witness Erickson following the same procedures—but always in fresh, creative expressions that are suited to the individuality of the subject. This consistency gives us confidence in our developing understanding of his approaches. In this section we see him once again attempting to facilitate the experience of hypnotic amnesia in order to cover and protect important hypnotherapeutic work from later interference by the patient's conscious mind. And once again we see him use a naturalistic metaphor that the subject has inevitably experienced: that of eating food, forgetting about having eaten, and having the food thoroughly digested in the meantime. By associating this common, natural body process with the subject's ongoing experience of trance, Erickson can hopefully facilitate an amnesia for the hypnotherapeutic work as natural as one's amnesia for eating. Erickson's rationale for using hypnotic amnesia and indirect suggestion is summarized in the following statement:[27]

> The practical problem of coping with the bridging associations between trance and waking states takes us directly to Erickson's utilization of amnesia to facilitate the effectiveness of hypnotherapeutic suggestion. As implied in our earlier discussion of the superiority of indirect over directly administered suggestions, the basic problem of securing reliable results from suggestions is to "protect" them from the doubting, debating, and potentially negating effects of the patient's conscious sets and attitudes. Patients are patients because of the erroneous and rigid sets that govern their maladaptive behavior. By administering suggestions indirectly so they are not recognized by consciousness, the suggestions are able to enter the patient's preconscious and/or unconscious and are there utilized in an optimal manner for the patient's overall development. Hypnotic amnesia is thus a convenient approach for coping with consciousness and protecting therapeutic suggestions from the limitations of the patient's conscious sets. Hypnotic amnesia effectively breaks the bridging associations between the trance and waking situation and thus seals hypnotic suggestions from the potentially negating effects of the patient's conscious attitudes. (p. 90)

Notice, too, that as in previous sections Erickson is being consistent in directing his indirect suggestions for amnesia to both rational and non-rational processes: the analogical framework engages the non-rational or right-hemispheric processes of the subject, while his use of truisms about digestion engage the subject's rational, left-hemispheric processes.

Therapeutic Analogies

Ratifying Trance and Hypnotic Amnesia for the Skeptical Scientific Mind

E: A friend of mine who is tremendously interested in research never knows if he has eaten. You can ask him, "Did you have lunch?", "Did you have dinner?" And he looks at you with that simple wonderment and says, "I must have—I'm not hungry—I'm just interested in this project." He must have eaten—he's not hungry. And yet on a Sunday he can eat his dinner with you, and comment on it afterwards, and really enjoy thinking about it, and really speculate on what he will have for dinner next Sunday. He doesn't have to remember that he ate so many calories to enable him to do so much work. As for whatever conscious curiosity you may have, you can find out how to satisfy that curiosity because your unconscious mind will enable you to do it in its own way. [Pause] Just as a doctor not so long ago wanted to be put into a trance, and wanted me to prove that he was in the trance. And I tried to persuade him to let his unconscious prove it to him... * but his unconscious was... And so he regretted that I did not put him in a trance, expressed his regrets to me, and watched me make certain notations in my notebook. Then a month later he wrote me a letter stating that he [had intended to] write me a letter, but he had put it off until this day. And then for some inner reason it seemed to be the only day to write the letter. And after he had written the letter I showed him my notebook. In my notebook was a statement that he would write the letter on a certain day; that he would use certain words; that he would

*Editors' Note: Ellipsis points indicate inaudible words.

express certain ideas. And the use of certain words and certain ideas would be rather unusual and out of keeping with his thinking. For example he used the word *fingers* when he really meant the word *hand*. [Pause] And he included in the letter half a dozen insults to my intelligence—seemingly insults. He labeled a piece of paper so that I would know which was the right side of the paper, which was the top side, which was the left side, which was the bottom—in spite of the fact that it was a sheet of paper on which there was writing, he still had to label it *right, left, top, bottom*. And anybody would know the right hand of a sheet of paper on which the English language is written. And if you know the right-hand side you certainly know the left-hand side; and if you can read, you certainly know which is the top and which is the bottom. But it was all beautifully labeled so that I was sure to read that sheet. And yet it was not an insult but *the carrying out of hypnotic behavior without his conscious knowledge.* It took him a whole month to do it, but it was beautifully done.

> ER: This therapeutic analogy of how Erickson ratified the existence of trance or unconscious effects on a professional colleague helps the skeptical, scientific portion of the subject's mind learn how to accept and even self-facilitate the experience of therapeutic trance. The hubris of Western consciousness requires that each new age invent new rationales for understanding and accepting altered states. It seems to be a characteristic of Western consciousness that it has always wanted to believe that it really "runs the show." It does not want to accept the autonomy of the unconscious. The attitudes of modern academic psychiatry and psychology are no different than those of the ancient Greeks in this regard. Thus Erickson devoted a great deal of his creative energy to developing ever more subtle means of validating the experience of therapeutic trance for his colleagues, who were much more difficult as patients than the general public.[28]

Reframing Life Problems

Reinterpreting the Speech Problem as an Expression of Character and Meaningfulness: "This Crooked Nose"; A Hypothesis Regarding the Role of Reframing in Integrating Conscious and Unconscious Processes of Change

E: In the matter of your speech, the perfectionistic quality that you want is only that quality that is fitting for you as a person. And your perfectionism should come in your utilization of your energies in the way that permits you to achieve the real objects of your functioning.

[Long pause]

Just as you mentioned that a portrait has been prostituted to a mere semblance, *that you want the defects in the portrait to be portrayed so that it is really a portrait of what is there, not some meaningless thing* **about which the observer can say some meaningless thing.** *So should your speech be meaningful and without the over-corrections that you consciously think you should enforce upon your speech. Because your speech problem is essentially an expression of over-corrections and a failure to accept the realities.* **A person's crooked nose may be the most meaningful feature of the face, and a portrait that shows a straight nose robs that picture of all its meaning. That crooked nose on the face does the breathing and expresses the character of the face.**

> ER: Only now—after a climax of therapeutic activation, floods of memories, and presumed hypnotic amnesia—does Erickson introduce a reframing of the subject's speech problem. Moreover, this reframing is in terms that the subject must find particularly meaningful, since it is associated with his highest levels of artistic sensibility: his sensitivity to the meaningfulness and character of portraits.

293

Why does this important reframe which deals with the basic speech problem come in now, only *after* the heightened phase of unconscious mental activity is over? Since the essence of the hypnotherapeutic process for Erickson was in this heightened state of unconscious activation—which by now has been covered at lease partially by amnesia—this process of reframing that follows must have another purpose. What can that purpose be? Can reframing simply be a way of restructuring *conscious* attitudes?! *The reframe is a way of helping the patient reorganize his conscious attitudes in a manner that corresponds with and supports "that reassociation and reorganization of ideas, understandings, and memories so essential for an actual cure" that was done by the autonomous unconscious during its period of heightened activation.* A good reframe usually has a particularly delightful quality that immediately feels right and is readily accepted by the conscious mind. Perhaps the conscious mind receives it so readily because the unconscious is already fermenting with it. Conscious and unconscious processes are thus mutually reinforced and can continue supporting one another through the new therapeutic associative network that is formed between them.

Another Therapeutic Analogy

Indirectly Relating the Speech Problem to Issues of Conformity and the Integrity of the Individual

E: Conformity to others seems to be such a nice thing, but it robs you of your integrity as an individual. And neither should you go all out to be non-conformist in everything. To be a non-conformist in dress does not mean that the non-conformity in itself should be the goal. A non-conformity in dress should relate to the self as an individual, and only to the self, and not be a means of using the non-conformity in dress for hitting other people in the eye. Just because the Texan dislikes the Bostonian does not mean that he must

exaggerate the Texas accent, nor should he try to assume a Bostonian accent. He should speak without saying a... of accent that he would use speaking in Texas to Texas friends—no more, no less. And he should speak to the Bostonian as he would his Texas friends, but for him to exaggerate his accent to the Bostonian falsifies things. To assume the Bostonian accent falsifies things. He should be a natural non-conformist in speech in Boston, but simply an individual who doesn't conform, and who does not conform at purely an individual level. Because he *is* a Texan; he just happens to be in Boston. But he is still a Texan; therefore he is not *really* a non-conformist. He is an individualist—an individual from Texas in Boston. And he is being true to himself, and yet in speech the... of that mistaken effort to conform originally. The stammerer, the stutterer, tries to force his speech to fit that of others instead of using his speech *for* others and *for* himself.

> ER: Erickson obviously views the subject's problem with stuttering as related to a more basic issue of conformity and individualism. Erickson uses the therapeutic analogy of a Texan in Boston speaking with his natural Texas accent as an expression of his individuality, not as a tool of offense. It is, of course, no accident that this therapeutic analogy has to do with speech—the patient's primary problem area.

Awakening from Trance

An Associative Network of Posthypnotic Suggestions for Freedom and Self-Expression; Imbedded, Interspersed Suggestions for Symptom Relief

Now after arousal, neither you nor I will know what your unconscious is going to do. It may do things that I recognize, that Dr. H recognizes; it may do things that you recognize; or it may keep its own secrets thoroughly. The only thing that I want it to do, and will instruct it to do, is to take an infinite pride, a personal pride, an individual pride, in being able to go to sleep in a trance state whenever a suitable occasion arises; to have a feeling of competence in the ability to go into a trance state whenever the suitable occasion arises; a willingness and a pride in the manifesting of that ability. After you arouse I want you to have a sense of freedom—freedom to do and say things that [you don't] understand without fear, without repression, and without withholding; with merely an expectation of being understood better by yourself than you ever realized; better by us than you can expect. **Now you can take it easily and rouse up.** [Long pause]

ER: Even though Erickson has a strong hunch about the specific psychodynamic sources of the subject's stuttering, he seems to end this phase of the trance work with a generalized though highly supportive set of posthypnotic suggestions. It would be tempting to gloss over this posthypnotic network, viewing it simply as a set of vaguely positive suggestions of the usual sort that is typically offered. A more careful study, however, reveals an intricate structure of mutually supporting suggestions balancing freedom of expression with some highly specific and very important indirect suggestions:

E: Now after arousal, neither you nor I will know what your unconscious is going to do.

ER: This appears to be a non-directive, *carte blanche* suggestion for total freedom. But the implication is that the subject's unconscious will be in control, directing. This is tantamount to saying that after arousal an altered state will continue wherein the unconscious has more control over mental life and behavior. The subject may think he is being told to awaken, but in fact he is being indirectly instructed to continue a special state of therapeutic responsiveness.

E: It may do things that I recognize, that Dr. H recognizes; it may do things that you recognize; or it may keep its own secrets thoroughly.

ER: That is a really fail-safe suggestion! It is almost a parody of the open-ended suggestion covering all possibilities of response, such that whatever the subject experiences is in rapport with Erickson and therefore reinforcing of whatever else Erickson says. But note that it is a natural continuation of the previous sentence that indirectly suggests that a special state of therapeutic responsiveness will continue. In this special state the therapeutic responses associated with Erickson, Dr. H, or the subject's own conscious-unconscious, now have a freedom to express themselves—but even if they do not, it will be of therapeutic value for the unconscious to "keep its own secrets thoroughly"! *Secrets* is a very special word in our culture. By the mere mention of *secrets* at this point Erickson is ideodynamically touching upon and utilizing the motivating energy of whatever inner psychodynamics the subject is most involved with to reinforce this final network of posthypnotic suggestions.

E: The only thing that I want it to do, and will instruct it to do, is to take an infinite pride, a personal pride, an individual pride, in being able to go to sleep in a trance state whenever a suitable occasion arises; to have a feeling of competence in the ability to go into a trance state whenever the suitable occasion arises; a willingness and a pride in the manifesting of that ability.

ER: Ah-ha—a nice, though apparently convoluted, direct suggestion at last! It must come as a relief to hear something so definitely supportive and upbeat that one can do. So refreshing might it be to hear these brightly direct suggestions that one does not quite realize their implications: (1) that Erickson and the therapeutic values he represents will be associated and ideodynamically activated whenever the subject does "go to sleep in a trance state whenever a suitable occasion arises"; and (2) that this therapeutic activation is now associated with "infinite *pride*, a personal *pride*, an individual *pride* ... a feeling of competence ... a willingness and a *pride* in the manifesting of that ability."

As Erickson might say with a slight, sly grin, that is an awfully great amount of therapeutic *pride* to stuff into one sentence!

E: After you arouse I want you to have a sense of freedom—freedom to do and say things that [you don't] understand without fear, without repressing, and without withholding; with merely an expectation of being understood better by yourself than you ever realized; better by us than you can expect.

ER: Phew! All that freedom without understanding, fear, repressing, or withholding. Is it possible? Is it contradictory? Who can digest such a cognitively and emotionally overloaded suggestion? Perhaps that is the meaning in Erickson's method. In any case it is reinforced positively with "an expectation of being understood better by yourself than you ever realized; better by us than you can expect." This ending focuses on a positive "expectation" of being understood.

As a final example of how subtle these suggestions can be, I must ask you, dear reader, if you noticed how blithely Erickson just gave the subject an imbedded, interspersed suggestion to overcome his stuttering?! Erickson's words flow out in such seeming cliches at times, but did you notice the significance of "freedom to do and *say* things ..."?

Some aspects of this associative network of posthypnotic suggestions are diagrammed in Figure 4.*

---

*Editors' Note: At this point the tape continues with interaction between Dr. Erickson and the subject. Unfortunately the editors were not able to include it due to time limitations on the accompanying audio cassette. The tape is on file at The Milton H. Erickson Foundation, 3606 North 24th Street, Phoenix, Arizona 85016.

Diagramming Associative Networks of Posthypnotic Suggestions

SYMPTOM RELIEF

Non-conformity; individualism; individual speech accents & idiosyncracies

FREEDOM ⟷ UNCONSCIOUS has control, free choice & secrets ⟷ SELF-EXPRESSION

To do and say things without fear, without repression, without withholding

Continue a special state of therapeutic response

Expectation of better self-understanding

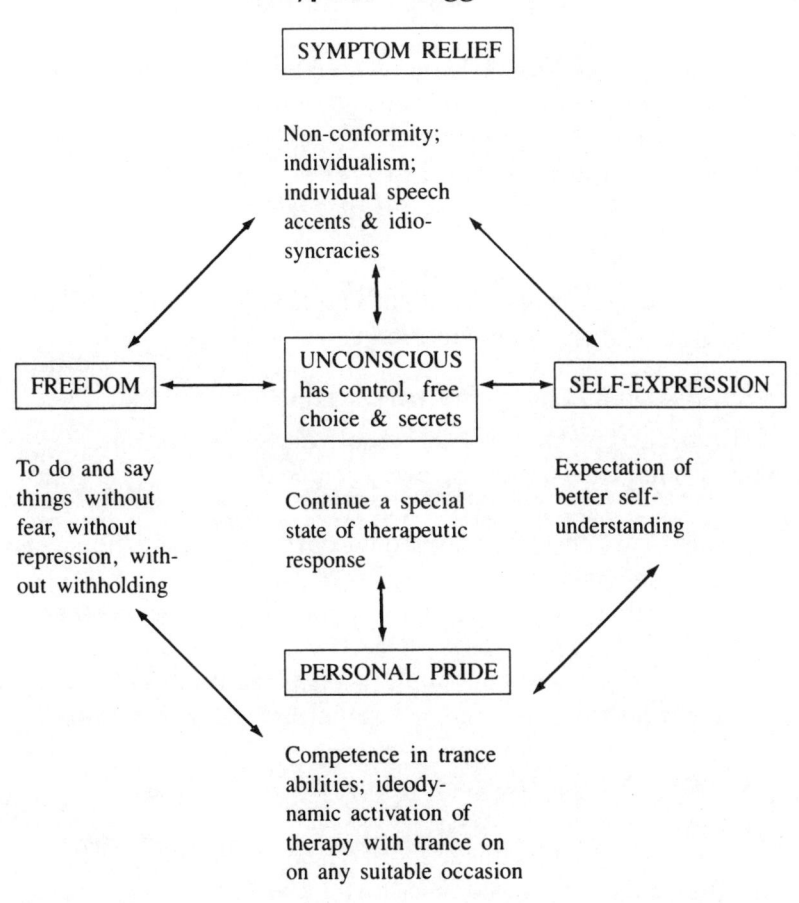

PERSONAL PRIDE

Competence in trance abilities; ideodynamic activation of therapy with trance on on any suitable occasion

Figure 4: Ratifying trance with an associative network of posthypnotic suggestions that are all mutually reinforcing and supportive of therapeutic possibilities in Section IV.

REFERENCES

Part I

1. See *Hypnotherapy* for further examples of the dynamics of shifting frames of reference in therapy.
2. For further illustrations of therapeutic double binds, see "Varieties of Double Bind" in Volume I of *Collected Papers* (pp. 412–429).
3. See *Hypnotherapy* for a discussion of this principle.
4. See Erickson's papers on the use of psychological shock and surprise in transforming self-image and identity, in Section IX of Volume IV, *Collected Papers*.
5. See "The Indirect Forms of Suggestion" in Volume I of *Collected Papers*, pp. 452–477.
6. See Rossi's discussion, "Ericksonian Hypnotherapy Now and in the Future," In J. Zeig (Ed.), *Ericksonian Approaches to Hypnosis and Psychotherapy* (New York: Brunner/Mazel, 1984); and J. L. McGaugh's article, "Preserving the Presence of the Past: Hormonal Influences on Memory Storage," in *American Psychologist* (1983, *38*, 161–174).
7. See "Hypnosis and Ultradian Cycles: A New State(s) Theory of Hypnosis?", written by Ernest Rossi. *The American Journal of Clinical Hypnosis*, 1982, *25* (1), 21–32.
8. See "The Reverse Set to Facilitate Hypnotic Induction" in *Experiencing Hypnosis* (pp. 154–180), for a detailed, verbatim video tape with commentary that provides an informative illustration of how Erickson utilized a specific mental mechanism to facilitate trance induction.

9. See "The Indirect Forms of Suggestion" in Volume I of *Collected Papers* (pp. 452–477).
10. Erickson presented this case as an example of indirect suggestion for amnesia in his paper, "The Problem of Amnesia in Waking and Hypnotic States" (Volume III of *Collected Papers*, pp. 58–70). This case is also a dramatic example of what Rossi later conceptualized as a form of *state-bound hypnotic amnesia*, in "Varieties of Hypnotic Amnesia" (Volume III of *Collected Papers*, pp. 71–90). The personal sources of this approach to amnesia can be found in one of Erickson's childhood experiences. He discovered that he would sometimes forget parts of a poem he had memorized earlier while sitting up in a tree—but would be able to recall the entire poem once he climbed back up the same tree!
11. These psychophysiological characteristics of the common everyday trance as a form of autohypnosis are outlined in detail in "Altered States of Consciousness in Everyday Life: The Ultradian Rhythms," by Ernest Rossi. In B. Wolman (Ed.), *The Handbook of Altered States of Consciousness* (New York: Van Nostrand, 1984).
12. See Section IV in Volume I of *Collected Papers*.
13. See "The Indirect Forms of Suggestion," in Volume I of *Collected Papers* (pp. 452–477).
14. For further illustrations of this concept, see *Hypnotic Realities* (pp. 103–104) and Volume I of *Collected Papers* (pp. 120–121).
15. See "Two-Level Communication and the Microdynamics of Trance and Suggestion" in Volume I of *Collected Papers* (pp. 430–451).
16. See Section II in *Experiencing Hypnosis* for a detailed presentation of Erickson's approaches to catalepsy.
17. See Andre Weitzenhoffer's discussion of this phenomenon in his book, *General Techniques of Hypnotism* (New York: Grune & Stratton), 1957.
18. See "The 'Surprise' and 'My-Friend-John' Techniques of Hypnosis: Minimal Cues and Natural Field Experimenta-

tion," in Volume I of *Collected Papers* (pp. 340–359) for more detailed illustrations of this approach.
19. See Section VIII of Volume IV in *Collected Papers*, "Self-Exploration in the Hypnotic State."
20. See the Index entries under "Minimal cues" in Volumes I and II of *Collected Papers* for further discussion of this topic.
21. See Section II in *Experiencing Hypnosis* for a detailed exposition on this hand levitation approach.
22. See Index listings in the four volumes of *Collected Papers* under the headings of "Experiential," "Experiential knowledge," and "Experiential learning."
23. See Section VII in Vol. IV of *Collected Papers*, "Sexual Problems: Hypnotherapeutic Reorientations to Emotional Satisfaction," for a great variety of examples of Erickson's approaches to shifting frames of reference (reframing).

Part II

1. This is an example of what Erickson and Rossi later conceptualized as the *conscious-unconscious double bind*. See "Varieties of Double Bind," in Volume I of *Collected Papers* (pp. 412–429).
2. This is a clear example of associating a suggestion—*Your unconscious will listen to what I say*—with a behavioral inevitability: *that their minds will wander*. For a discussion of this approach, see Chapter 4 in *Hypnotherapy*.
3. See Section II of *Experiencing Hypnosis* for further discussion and illustration of this approach (in particular, see pages 41–47).
4. See index headings under "Frames of reference" in *Hypnotherapy*. See also *Ericksonian Approaches to Hypnosis and Psychotherapy*, J. Zeig (Ed.). New York: Brunner/Mazel, 1982; and *Reframing: Neuro-Linguistic Programming and the Transformation of Meaning*, written by R. Bandler and J. Grinder (Moab, Utah: Real People Press), 1982.

5. See "Two-Level Communication and the Microdynamics of Trance and Suggestion," in Volume I of *Collected Papers* (pp. 430–451).
6. See "Hypnotic Investigation of Psychosomatic Phenomena: Psychosomatic Interrelationships Studied by Experimental Hypnosis," in Volume II of *Collected Paper,* pp. 145–156.
7. Presumably Erickson's comments on anesthetized responsiveness were in response to Cheek's presentation of his paper, "Unconscious Perception of Meaningful Sounds During Surgical Anesthesia as Revealed in Hypnosis," published in 1959 by *The American Journal of Clinical Hypnosis* (*1*, 103–113).

PART III

1. For additional applications of the My-Friend-John Technique, see "The 'Surprise' and 'My-Friend-John' Technique of Hypnosis: Minimal Cues and Natural Field Experimentation," in Vol. I of *Collected Papers*, pp. 340–359.
2. See the papers in Section IV on "Time Distortion" in Vol. II of *Collected Papers*.
3. See Robert Ader (Ed.), *Psychoneuroimmunology* (New York: Academic Press), 1982.
4. There is a long and important history of observation and speculation regarding the role of eyeball and eyelid movements during hypnotic induction and trance. Unfortunately, however, there is relatively little experimental research in this area. A recent computer search of psychological abstracts offered the following three papers, each of which contains findings of observational interest for clinicians:

   Gur, R., & Reyher, J. Relationships Between Style of Hypnotic Induction and Direction of Lateral Eye Movements. *The Journal of Abnormal Psychology*, 1973, *82*(3), 499–505.

   Tebecis, A., & Provins, K. Hypnosis and Eye Movements. *Biological Psychology*, 1975, *3*(1), 31–47.

Weitzenhoffer, A. Ocular Changes Associated with Passive Hypnotic Behavior. *The American Journal of Clinical Hypnosis*, 1971, *14*(2), 102–121.

A fourth helpful reference is a book-length treatment of the use and diagnostic significance of eye roll in hypnosis and personality type:

Spiegel, H., & Spiegel, D. *Trance and Treatment*. New York: Basic Books, 1978.

The recognition of eye movements as a part of the process of remembering was later greatly elaborated into the concept of "assessing cues" as part of the *Neuro-Linguistic Programming* (NLP) approach to hypnotherapy:

Dilts, R., Grinder, J., Bandler, R., DeLozier, J., & Cameron-Bandler, L. *Neuro-Linguistic Programming. I.* Cupertino, Calif.: Meta Publications, 1979.

Unfortunately this work has had no experimental validation that the editors were able to locate at this time.

PART IV

1. See Section IV of *Experiencing Hypnosis*, "The Experiential Learning of Trance by the Skeptical Mind," (pp. 181–257) for an extensive illustration of this process.
2. See *Experiencing Hypnosis* for a detailed discussion of how to evoke and utilize arm catalepsies in hypnotherapy.
3. See "Further Experimental Investigation of Hypnosis: Hypnotic and Nonhypnotic Realities," in Volume I of *Collected Papers* (pp. 18–82). See also the section on literalism in Volume III of *Collected Papers* (pp. 91–101).

PART V

1. See "Two-Level Communication and the Microdynamics of Trance Induction and Suggestion," Volume I, *Collected Papers* (pp. 430–451).
2. In *Hypnotherapy*.

3. For a discussion of ultradian cycles see "Altered States of Consciousness in Everyday Life: the Ultradian Rhythms," by Ernest Rossi. In B. Wolman (Ed.), *The Handbook of Altered States of Consciousness* (New York: Van Nostrand, 1984).
4. See Ernest Hilgard's, *Divided Consciousness: Multiple Controls in Human Thought and Action* (New York: Wiley & Sons, 1977), for experimental research documenting the "hidden observer" during hypnosis.
5. This is based on one of the oldest ideas in the history of hypnosis regarding the essence of hypnotic suggestibility. Bernheim formulated it as follows:
> The one thing certain is, that a peculiar *aptitude for transforming the idea received into acts* exists in hypnotized subjects who are susceptible to suggestion...
> In the hypnotized subject... the transformation of thought into action, sensation, movement, or vision is so quickly and so actively accomplished that the intellectual inhibition [by conscious intentionality] has not time to act.

From *Suggestive Therapeutics: A Treatise on the Nature and Uses of Hypnotism* (Westport, Conn.: Associated Booksellers, 1957; originally published by Putnam, New York, 1886, translated by C. A. Herter), p 137.
6. From *The Structure and Dynamics of the Psyche*, Volume 8 of *The Collected Works of C. G. Jung*. Edited by H. Read, M. Fordham, & G. Adler, Bollingen Series 20 (New York: Pantheon Books), 1960, p. 74.
7. See the listings under *Utilization* in the Indexes of the four volumes of *Collected Papers* and the three Erickson-Rossi volumes.
8. Otto Rank's books, *Art and the Artist* (New York: Knopf, 1932) and *The Myth of the Birth of the Hero and Other Writings* (New York: Vintage, 1959), contain some of the more original insights into this view of symptoms as frustrated forms of creativity.
9. See "The Autohypnotic Experiences of Milton H. Erick-

son" in Volume I of *Collected Papers* (pp. 108–132), and "Milton H. Erickson: A Biographical Sketch" in *Healing in Hypnosis,* which is Volume I of this series (pp. 1 -59; in particular, pp. 10–14).
10. See Bateson's workshop in M. Berger (Ed.), *Beyond the Double Bind* (New York: Brunner/Mazel, 1978).
11. For a detailed explication of the ultradian hypothesis and the subtle behavioral indications of our daily rhythms of shifting consciousness, see Ernest Rossi's "Altered States of Consciousness in Everyday Life: The Ultradian Rhythms." In B. Wolman (Ed.), *The Handbook of Altered States of Consciousness* (New York: Van Nostrand, 1984).
12. From "Hypnotic Psychotherapy," in Volume IV of *Collected Papers* (pp. 35–48).
13. See "Clinical and Experimental Trance: Hypnotic Training and Time Required for Their Development," in Volume II of *Collected Papers* (pp. 301–306).
14. See R. Carnap, *The Logical System of Language* (Patterson, New Jersey: Littlefield, Adams Co., 1959), and A. Whitehead and B. Russell, *Principia Mathematica* (2nd edition, Cambridge: University Press, 1925).
15. This article can be found in Volume I of *Collected Papers,* pp. 533–535.
16. See "Concerning the Nature and Character of Posthypnotic Behavior," in Volume I of *Collected Papers* (pp. 381–411).
17. See Volume III of *Collected Papers.* In particular, see Section 1 on "Amnesia" and Section 5 on "Mental Mechanisms" in Part II, "Psychodynamic Processes: Hypnotic Approaches to the Unconscious."
18. See "Two-Level Communication and the Microdynamics of Trance and Suggestion" in Volume I of *Collected Papers* (pp. 430–451).
19. See "Possible Detrimental Effects of Experimental Hypnosis" (in Volume I of *Collected Papers,* pp. 493–497), in which Erickson reported in regard to the trance state: "Far from making them [the subjects] hypersuggestible, it was found necessary to deal very gingerly with them to keep

from losing their cooperation, and it was often felt that they developed a compensatory negativism toward the hypnotist to offset any increased suggestibility" (p. 495).
20. See E. H. Hess, B. K. Rhoades, A. W. Hodges, and E. S. Abbott, Jr., "An Inexpensive, Nondedicated, Automated Pupillometric Measurement System." *Perceptual & Motor Skills*, 1982, *54*(1), 235–241.
21. Quoted from Volume IV of *Collected Papers*, pp. 35–48.
22. See the many case examples in *Hypnotherapy* illustrating this approach.
23. From *Hypnotherapy*, p. 7.
24. From *Hypnotic Realities*, p. 311.
25. See J.L. McGaugh's article, "Preserving the Presence of the Past: Hormonal Influences on Memory Storage." *American Psychologist*, 1983, *38*(2), pp. 161–174.
26. See *Hypnotic Realities, Hypnotherapy,* and *Experiencing Hypnosis* for a variety of approaches to ratifying therapeutic trance.
27. Quoted from "Varieties of Hypnotic Anmesia," Volume III of *Collected Papers*, pp. 71–90.
28. See "The Experiential Learning of Trance by the Skeptical Mind" in *Experiencing Hypnosis* for one of Erickson's more subtle appoaches to training a young psychiatrist to experience trance (pp. 181–257).

BIBLIOGRAPHY

Ader, R. *Psychoneuroimmunology.* New York: Academic Press, 1982.

Bandler, R., & Grinder, J. *Reframing: Neuro-Linguistic Programming and the Transformation of Meaning.* Moab, Utah: Real People Press, 1982.

Bateson, G. "Addendum 1: Bateson Workshop." In M. Berger (Ed.), *Beyond the Double Bind.* New York: Brunner/Mazel, 1978 (pp. 197–230).

Carnap, R. *The Logical System of Language.* Paterson, New Jersey: Littlefield, Adams Co., 1959.

Cheek, D. Unconscious Perception of Meaningful Sounds During Surgical Anesthesia as Revealed in Hypnosis. *The American Journal of Clinical Hypnosis*, 1959, *1*, 103–113.

Dilts, R., Grinder, J., Bandler, R., Delozier, J., & Cameron-Bandler, L. *Neuro-Linguistic Programming, I.* Cupertino, Calif.: Meta Publications, 1979.

Erickson, M. *The Collected Papers of Milton H. Erickson on Hypnosis (4 vols.).* Edited by Ernest Rossi. New York: Irvington Publishers, 1980.
- Volume I: *The Nature of Hypnosis and Suggestion*
- Volume II: *Hypnotic Alteration of Sensory, Perceptual, and Psychophysical Processes*
- Volume III: *Hypnotic Alteration of Psychodynamic Processes*
- Volume IV: *Innovative Hypnotherapy*

Erickson, M., Rossi, E., & Rossi, S. *Hypnotic Realities.* New York: Irvington, 1976.

Erickson, M., & Rossi, E. *Hypnotherapy: An Exploratory Casebook.* New York: Irvington, 1969.

Erickson, M., & Rossi, E. *Experiencing Hypnosis.* New York: Irvington, 1981.

Gur, R., & Reyher, J. Relationships Between Style of Hypnotic Induction and Direction of Lateral Eye Movements. *The American Journal of Clinical Hypnosis,* 1973, *16*(3), 499–505.

Hess, E.H., Rhoades, B.K., Hodges, A.W., & Abbott, E.S. An Inexpensive, Nondedicated, Automated Pupillometric Measurement System. *Perceptual & Motor Skills,* 1982, *54*(1), 235–241.

Hilgard, E. *Divided Consciousness: Multiple Controls in Human Thought and Action.* New York: Wiley & Sons, 1977.

Jung, C. *The Structure and Dynamics of the Psyche.* Volume 8 of *The Collected Works of C. G. Jung,* edited by H. Read, M. Fordham, & G. Adler. New York: Pantheon Books, 1960.

McGaugh, J. Preserving the Presence of the Past: Hormonal Influences on Memory Storage. *American Psychologist,* 1983, *38*(2), 161–174.

Rank, O. *Art and the Artist.* New York: Knopf, 1932.

Rank, O. *The Myth of the Birth of the Hero and Other Writings.* New York: Vintage, 1959.

Rossi, E. *Dreams and the Growth of Personality.* New York: Pergamon, 1972.

Rossi, E. Hypnosis and Ultradian Cycles: A New State(s) Theory of Hypnosis? *The American Journal of Clinical Hypnosis,* 1982, *25,* 21–32.

Rossi, E. Altered States of Consciousness in Everyday Life: The Ultradian Rhythms. In B. Wolman (Ed.), *The Handbook of Altered States of Consciousness.* New York: Van Nostrand, 1984.

Rossi, E., Ryan, M., & Sharp, F. (Eds.) *Healing in Hypnosis: The Seminars, Workshops, and Lectures of Milton H. Erickson* (Vol. I). New York: Irvington, 1983.

Spiegel, H., & Spiegel, D. *Trance and Treatment.* New York: Basic Books, 1978.

Tebecis, A., & Provins, K. Hypnosis and Eye Movements. *Biological Psychology,* 1975, *3*(1), 31–47.
Watzlawick, P., Weakland, J., & Fisch, R. *Change: Principles of Problem Formation and Problem Resolution.* New York: W. W. Norton, 1974.
Weitzenhoffer, A. *General Techniques of Hypnotism.* New York: Grune & Stratton, 1957.
Weitzenhoffer, A. Ocular Changes Associated with Passive Hypnotic Behavior. *The American Journal of Clinical Hypnosis,* 1971, *14*(2), 102–121.
Whitehead, A., & Russell, B. *Principia Mathematica* (2nd edition). Cambridge: University Press, 1925.
Zeig, J. (Ed.) *Ericksonian Approaches to Hypnosis and Psychotherapy.* New York: Brunner/Mazel, 1984.

INDEX

Abraham, Karl xiv
Age regression 99, 133
All possibilities of
  response 178, 253
Allan (Erickson) 10, 48
Altered (state)
  everyday life and **261f**
  experience of 258
  involuntary behavior and 238
  phenomenological issues and
    269f
  sensory-perceptual 258
Ambivalence
  time binding choice and 13
American Society of Clinical
    Hypnosis (ASCH)
  authoritarian views and 173
  smoking and 173
Amnesia (hypnotic) 105, 226,
    285
  desirability of 126
  everyday life 158
  facilitating 78, 90, 99, **289f**
  implication and 62
  indirect 59, 62

source 273
teaching 156
Analysis
  Erickson's view of **168, 209**
  Freudian xiv
  past and **209**
  reframing 168
  symptom change and 168
Analyst
  transference and **251**
Anesthesia (analgesia) 105, 164,
    228
  dental 33f, 178
  discussed 90
  Erickson's experiments
    with 184
  ideodynamic 16
  localized 122
  obstetrical 178
  total body 80, 155
Anne 54
Anxiety
  approaches to 7
  control of 14
  responses 87

Appetite control 47
Archetypal collective
    unconscious xiv
Arithmetic progression
    trance deepening 58
    treating insomnia 118
Associative (associational)
        (networks) 109, **245f**, **264**,
        295f
    bridging 290
    diagramming **255f**, **298f**
    early learning sets **287**
    gaps 105
    motivation **287**
    posthypnotic **298f**
    real memories **261f**
Aston, Ted 204
Attention
    edge of 153
    fixating 14, 38, 142, 149,
        154, 170
    focusing 150, 152, 154
    hypnotic **170**
    redirecting 146
    shifting 7, 170
    unconscious 154
    wide open 142, 149
Attitude
    renewal 251
    reorganizing **294f**
Audience hypnotic
    induction 130
Audition 66
Authoritarian 173
Autohypnosis (autohypnotic) 47,
        52, 54
    hallucinated "Joe"
        induction 53, 93
    learning 53, 63
    posthypnotic suggestions
        for 72, 130

techniques 62, 193
unconscious and 63
utilizing 64
Automatic
    movement 59
    writing 90
Autonomic nervous system **246**
Autonomous (*See also*
        Unconscious)
    activity **287f**
    habits 38
    unconscious 294
Awareness **223f**
    hypnosis and **223f**
    levels of **200f**
    receptivity and 223
    special states and **223f**

B, Dr. 187
Bateson, G. 267f, 271
Baudoin, 90
Behavior(al)
    cues **276f**
    hyperactive 89
    inevitabilities 76, 144, 273
    manipulation 106
    purposive vs. non-purposive
    responsive **22**, **280f**
    utilization of 21
Bernice 89f, 115f
Betty Alice (Erickson) 10
Binds **12**, 177
Birth control 198
Blackboard technique 212
Bladder urgency 27
Blindness
    inducing hypnotic 66
Blood flow control 121
Body
    experiential learning
        & knowledge 121

Brody, Dr. 44, 55, 90

"Calloused nerves" 129
Cancer (*See also* Pain)
  components of 24
  examples of 27f
  pain control in **24f, 27f,** 158, 163, 166, 174
  time distortion for 24
Case examples and stories
  Allan 10, 48
  Betty Alice 10
  blocked artist 52
  Dr. L 24
  MHE's creative comics 51
  MHE's smoking 172
  MHE's unfinished manuscript 50
  Mrs. Erickson's forgotten task 47
  Robert's stitches 7
  Robert's truck accident 123
  Twenty-five-cent experiment 64
  "Which knife to use?" 205
Catalepsy (cataleptic) (*See also* Ideomotor)
  confusion in 85
  discussed 82
  examples of 80, 87, 94, 98, 226, 239
  hand 87
  hypnosis and 202f
  inducing 154
  muscle tonus and 154
  suspension 277
  tactile suggestions for 111, 155
  trance indicator 112

Catharsis 119
Cheek, D. 187
Children('s) (childhood)
  control 182
  fixating attention 149
  hyperactive 210
  nightmares 123
  urinary problem 191
Choice
  double binds and **12**
  free **12f**
  time binding 13
Climax (hypnotherapeutic)
  facilitating **285f**
  therapeutic activation 293
Comfort 234
Common Everyday Trance (*See also* Hypnosis) **256f, 264**
  cataleptic suspension as 277
  ultradian hypothesis and **268f**
Communicating (*See also* Ideas)
  ideas **178**
  metalevels **271**
Compound suggestions 19, 60
Compulsions 127
Conditioning
  bruxism 40
  response 111
Confidence 125
Confusion
  examples of 77, **235f**
  in catalepsy 85
  in hand levitation 152
  overcoming pin phobia 107
Conscious (mind) 50, 119
  anesthesia 184
  expanding xiii
  hypnosis **247f**
  intentionality **247**
  irrelevance of 143
  resistance labeling **266f**

Conscious and unconscious
   conflict 266
   double bind 143, **266f**
   explaining 143
   insight and xiv
   integrating 293
   relations between **119f, 193f**
   separating 144
   uniting **251**
Contingent suggestions 71, 85, 91, 174, 175, 187, 188, 238, 267
Control **22**
   goal-directed behavior **22**
   reframing and 38
   utilizing 184
Cooperation via ideas 15
Coulton, Dr. 205
Creative (creativity) (receptive approach)
   facilitating xiii, **238, 249**
   hypnosis **238**
   possibilities 249
   self 259
   vs. democratic **174**
Cues
   minimal 69, 72
   subtle 87
Cure 104
   hypnosis and **171**
   psychodynamics of 208f
   "reassociation and reorganization" **269f, 287f**

Deafness (hypnotic) 228
Defenses 94
Democratic
   hypnosis and **173f**
Dentistry (dental)
   anesthesia 33, 122
   comfortable dentures 17

contraindications 124
hyperasthesia 33
implication facilitating 21
indirect ideodynamic focusing in 15
indirect induction in 14
posthypnotic suggestion in 6
time binds 10
Depotentiating
   conflict 267
   conscious attitudes 173
   examples of 104, 173
   fear in hypnosis 18
   learned limitations 252f, **256**
   obsessive compulsive 205
   phobic behavior 205
   resistance 267
Developmental shifts 287
Diet 47
Direct approach
   smoking control 172
Discovery 1, 37
Dissociation (dissociating)
   altered states and 68
   cancer pain 27
   dreams 164
   examples of 70, 166, **252f**
   facilitating 99
   "goal-defined" 90
   pain control 27
   prolonging 181
   somnambulistic 27, 31
   thinking and doing 55
   trance indicator, as 112
Distraction 105, 146, 149, 154, 156, 167
   fixating attention 14
   for pain 155, 176
Double bind **12**
   conscious-unconscious 143, **266f**

examples of **43, 57, 83,** 214, 217
multiple choice and 212
questions 43, **57,** 71
sensory-kinesthetic memories 212
therapeutic 189, 190
Doubt
  discharging 163
  evoking 141
Dreams
  experiential learning and 225
  external reality and **226f**
  hypnosis and 225
  memories and 226
  rhythms 246
  self-creation and **259f**
  therapeutic analogies 259
  utilizing 164, **225f**

Early learning sets **264, 287**
Edward and Jeanie 197f
Ego control 90
Energy
  constructive conversion of **279f**
  motivating 297
  rechanneling **283f**
Erickson, Milton
  personal and family history xv, 2, 7, 34, 50, 172f, 184f, 202, 260
Erickson, Mrs. (Elizabeth) 9, 47
Ethics in hypnosis 122
Expectancy (expectation)
  facilitating hypnotic response 75, 103
  pivotal role of **64**
  positive 18, 99
  versus direct suggestion 78

Experiential
  control and 38
  dream and 225
  learning **120f,** 180, 225
  life 280
  metaphor 289
  reassociating 280
  utilizing 225
  values 165
  variables 38
Exploration (hypnotic) 258
Eye closure
  ratification of trance 235
  suggestions for 92, 235

Facilitating (facilitation) (*See also* Utilizing)
  amnesia 78
  freedom to experience 10
  hallucination 94, 164
  learning and recall 44
  neuropsychophysiological responses 24
  new attitudes 17
  potentials **243f**
  relaxation 141
  response readiness 152, 153
Faith healing 103
False (fake)
  hypnotic response 239
  understanding 10
Family participation 177
Fear and anxiety 18, 19
Ferenczi, Sandor xiv
Fixation of attention 14, 39, 146
Forgetting (*See also* Amnesia) 126
Fractional approach 161, 163
Frames of reference xv, **189f, 200f**
Freedom **299**

Freud, S. xiv
Future perspective 195, 198, 199

Gale 122
Gaze 38
Generalization 146
Gorton, Bernie 134, 204
Group process
   creative hypnosis and 1, 62, **173f**
   hypnotherapy and 41
Growth xiv
Guilt
   indirect treatment of 207

Habit problems 20, 35, 39
   appetite control 47
   bruxism 39
   nontraumatic basis of 20
   reframing 38
   smoking 172
   thumbsucking 20
   tics 37
   transforming 41
Hallucination
   enhancing 219
   evoking 261
   experience **98,** 102, 164
   "hallucinated Joe" 53, 93
   mechanisms of 26
   "My-Friend-John" technique 194
   negative, training for 80
   self 99, 102
   "spontaneous" 94
   structured 220
   visual 109, 217
Hand levitation (*See also* Catalepsy, Ideomotor)
   examples of 71, 85, 258
   for trance deepening 58

inducing 111, 152, 154
   signaling 210
   technique 141
Harren, Dave 25
Head signaling 210
Headaches 118
Healing
   Erickson's theory of **269f**
   hypnotic 116
   natural 256
Hindsight 195, 199
Horney, Karen xiv
Humor
   in hypnosis 234
Hyperasthesia
   dental 33
   shifting 33
Hypersuggestibility 278
Hypnosis (hypnotic) (*See also* Trance) 140f, 146f, 148, 177, **223**
   advanced 195
   attention and 170
   audience 43f
   awareness and 223
   belief in 18
   cure and **171**
   degree of 146
   dental 124
   ethics in 122
   experiential learning and 200f
   goals 204
   group 62, 173
   inducing 161, 162
   interrelationships in 180
   language 32
   learning 122
   levels of awareness 200
   medical 150
   medication in 117
   nature of **223f**

neurodermatitis and 128
pain control 24, 27, 156,
  163, 164, 166, 174, 176
placebos in 117
positive expectancy in 18
reframing symptoms 167, **200**
stage 178, 273
successful 150
time in 151
treating compulsions 127
treating pruritis 129
without awareness 145
Hypnotic (trance) induction (*See also* Trance)
  audience 46, 130
  comparing induction and reinduction 139
  conversational 235
  developing 140
  hyperactive children and 210
  indirect 14, 23, 38, 104, 142
  resistance in 84
  successful 125
  three-stage 75
  via distraction 14
  via touch 14
  vicarious 176
Hypnotic phenomena
  defined **226**
  everyday basis of 228
  forms 283
  normal patterns of behavior **226f**
  spontaneous 264
Hypnotic Study Club 34
Hypnotherapists
  indivisuality of 216
  no magic 278
Hypnotherapy (hypnotherapeutic) (*See also* Hypnosis)
  activation 279, **184**

climax **279f, 285f**
enhancing probabilities **265**
essence **283f**, 198
failure 198
group 41
learning and 284
Hypothalamus
  limbic system and 202
Hysterectomy 199

Iatrogenic
  disease 104
  healing 104
  reinforcement 252
Ideas (*See also* Ideodynamic)
  facilitating denture wear 17
  hypnosis as 20, 140, 177
  presenting 15
  reassociate and reorganize 287, 269
Ideodynamic (processes) **68**
  comfort 67
  examples of 93, 249
  focusing 15, **16, 256**
  indirect 16
  motivating 297
  reinforcing **245**
  secrets 247
Ideomotor (movements)
  autonomous 52
  cues 210
  head 43, 87
  involuntary 74
  trance indicators 75
  trance induction 85
  validity of 210
Implication (implicative)
  control and 22
  examples of 19, 20f, 60, 62, 78, 166, 188

319

Implication (implicative) *(Cont'd)*
  facilitating responsiveness 94, 188
  overcoming pin phobia 107
  "proving" hypnotic pain reduction 27
  requests 187
  structuring 207
  unconscious 177, 267, 273
  work 273
Indirect (approaches)
  apposition of opposites 33
  cancer pain 174
  direct and 207
  examples of 19, 169, 207
  hypnotic techniques 14, 38, 133, 174, 235
  ideodynamic focusing 15
  patient reassurance 187
  posthypnotic suggestions 72
  smoking control 172
  suggestions 19, **283f**
  symptom correction 167, 170
  teaching 277
  therapeutic 251
  visualization 212
Individual (individuality) xiii, **238, 257f, 299**
  defined 43
  experience 259
  hypnotherapists as 216
  integrity of 294
  protecting 98
  trance states 204
Induction *(See also* Hypnotic induction)
  conversational 235
Inner search
  evoking 141, 150
  examples of 20, 173
  wondering and 257
Insight xiv

Insomnia 118
Investigating 172
Involuntary *(See also* Autonomous, Unconscious)
  tactile cues and 87
Inward focus *(See also* Unconscious) 238

Joe 53f, 76
Joke
  double bind and 268
Jung, Carl xiv, 250

Keat, Dr. 187
Kohler, W. xv

L, Dr. 25f
Language (linguistic)
  errors 139
  in hypnosis 32
  influence of 32
Law of Reversed Effects 87
Learned limitations **251f**
  depotentiating 252
Learning(s)
  altering 164
  autohypnosis 53, 72
  disabilities 182
  early sets 261
  experiential 180, **200f, 232f**
  facilitating 44, 46, 194
  indirect suggestions for 19
  relaxation and **284**
  sensory 166
  subjective 166
  unconscious **46f**
  verbalization 140
  without awareness 46
Life experiences *(See also* Learning)
  "reserve bank" 1
  Utilizing 1, **232f**

Life reframing **243f**
Literalism **240f**

Magic
  hand and eye 158
  no power **278**
  suggestions and **278**
Mann, Dr. 139
Margie 91f, 115f
Maslow, A. xv
Medication 117
Memory (*See also* Remembering)
  activation of 214
  "floods" 285
  image **260f**
  motor 219
  reality of mental life **259f**
  reassociating 280
  recall 223
  visual 282
Menstrual distress 3
Mental (mechanisms) 156
  activation of 255
  life speed of **286f**
Metalevel **267f**
  activating 270
  motivational **270f, 287**
  object level and 267
Metaphor
  childhood as 270
  concrete road 284
  experiential **288f**
  forgetting 289
  mythopoetic 282
  naturalistic 289
  "opening flower" 247, 256
  picture 259
  therapeutic 191
Microdynamics
  group 173
  of trance induction 85, 173

smoking and 173
Mind
  reading 105
  wandering 245, **256**
Minimal
  approaches 107
  cues 69, 72, 105, **276f**
Miraculous
  cures 103, 105
  power 280
Motivation **270f, 287**
  evoking 182, 297
  increasing 163
  symptom removal 118
  trance 238
Multiple levels
  of meaning 207
  of suggestion **275f**
Multiplicity
  choices 212
  suggestions **212**
Muscle
  catalepsy and 155f
  tonus 155f
"My-Friend-John"
  technique 194

Nash, Ogden 200
Naturalistic xiii
  approaches to trance **244f**
Negative
  discharging 220
  examples of 19, 20, 158, 220
  indirect suggestions for learning 19
  setting limits 163
Neurodermatitis 128
Neuroendocrinal (neurohormonal) **284**
  sensory responses and 26
Neuropsychophysiological
  examples of 24

Neuropsychophysiological *(Cont'd)*
  facilitating 24
  neurotransmitters 26
Neurotransmitters
  metaphor and 26
New
  frames of reference for old **200**
  receptivity to 219
Nightmares 123
Not knowing 67f, 71f, 75, 77, 94, 98, 172
  examples of 20, 208f, 235, 241, 256
  hypnotic learning and 201
  nature of cure **209**

Obesity 184, 189
Obsessive-compulsive 205
Observational abilities 276
Obstetrics
  anesthesia in 178
  facilitating suggestion in 21
Organic spasms 35

Pain
  approaches to 7, 55
  catalepsy and 155
  control 24f, 27f, **156f, 158f, 163f, 164f, 166f, 174f, 176f**
  organic component 24
  personality component 24
Paradoxical
  examples of 84, 207, **235f**
  questions 170
  response inhibition and 219
  suggestions 84, 116, 117, 207, 235
  voice tone 235
  wide awake 237
Parasympathetic (processes) 67f

Passive compliance **270f,** 287
Patients
  free expression 140
  participation 161, 174
  personal rights 122
  "triple-layered recognition" 151
  utilizing viewpoint 170
Paul 68f, 76
Pause
  hypnotherapeutic activation and **280f**
Perls, Fritz xv
Permission (permissive)
  in dissociation 181
  resistance and 253
  utilization and 173
Personal pride **299**
Personality
  cancer pain and 24
  disturbances 124
  free to express 216
  responsive to hypnosis **203f**
  total 279
Phenomenological
  altered states **269f**
  issues **269f**
  motivation and **270**
Phobia **205f**
  pin 107
Physiological (physical)
  altered 232
  contact 111
  control of 121, **229f**
  unconscious alteration of 232
  urinary urgency 192
Placebos 117
Positive
  indirect suggestions 19
Posthypnotic
  appetite control 47

322

associational network **299f**
behavioral inevitabilities
   and 273
covering all contingencies 3
curious 274f
demonstrated 76
dental 6
fail-safe **277**
freedom and 295
future autohypnotic
   experiences 130
future life changes 5
indirect 72
menstrual distress 3
rehearsal and 274
self-expression 295
suggestion 112, 287, **228f**, 295
trance 229
Potentials
   evoking **257f, 261f**
   facilitating **243f**
   highest **248f**, 256
   transference and **248f**
   unconscious **244**
Power 261
   hypersuggestibility and 278
   twentieth-century
      consciousness and 201
Premature ejaculation 190
Prescribing the symptom 117
   examples of 22, 85
Problem-solving **133f**
   creative 1
   personal 199
   psychodynamics of 208
   unconscious 51
Promise 187
Pruritis 129
Pseudo-orientation 195
Psychic phenomena 105

Psychological
   control of physiological
      functions 120
   interrelationships 156, 164
   problems xivf, **208f**
   reorientation 125, 128, 136
Psychoneuroimmunology 202
Psychophysiological
   control of 120
   dynamics in trance **246f**
   examples of 24
   responses **16**
   suggestion **16**
   ultradian 52, 67
   unconscious **16**
   utilizing 105
Psychosis 124
   catalepsy and 202
   schizophrenics vs.
      hypnosis 202
Psychosomatic processes (*See also* Psychophysiological)
   interrelationships of 180
Pupillary dilation
   conscious interest 276
   unconscious involvement 276

Questions
   and answers 116
   double bind 43, 57, 71
   evoking 148
   evoking catalepsy 112
   facilitating denture wear 17
   facilitating hypnotic
      response 75, 94
   facilitating visual
      hallucination 109
   for hand levitation 85
   moot 284
   paradoxical 170
   permissive 262

Questions *(Cont'd)*
   reframing symptoms 37f,
      167, 170f
   reviving original trance 23
   series **275**
   surprising 84
   wondering and **284**

Rank, Otto xiv
Rapport 253, 297
Raynaud's disease 229
Reality
   consensual
   memories and 259
Reassociation and
      reorganization **269, 287**
   ideas **287f**
Receptivity 80, 141, **223f**
   ideas as 223
   special states of 223
Reframing **xivf, 10, 38, 133f,**
      182, **200f, 288f, 243f,**
   altering entire picture **170f**
   childhood 271
   conscious and unconscious
      293f
   consensual reality 259
   distress 7, 10, 257, 271
   examples of 183, 205, **252f**
   hypothesis **293**
   inner experience xiv
   life **243f**
   life problems **293f**
   negativity 271
   new variables and 207
   nightmares 123
   obstinacy 270
   perfectionism 251, **255**, 271
   physiological functioning
      233f
   pruritis 129

psychological problems 38
reinterpretation and **205f**
sexual problems 125
shifting frames of
   reference 38
symptoms 167, 170
therapeutic analogies 255
thumbsucking 116
tics 37
Relationship in hypnosis 234
Relaxation 67
   catatonic 203
   dynamics of **246f**
   facilitating 141, 256
   muscle tension and **22**
Religious
   hypnosis and 174
Remembering (*See also*
      Memory)
   amnesia and 61
   desirability of 126
   operating room events 184
Reorganizing attitudes **294f**
Resistance
   accepting **218f**
   converting 69
   discharging **266f**
   examples of 17, 71, 89, 218
   minimal cues of 72
   overcoming 176, 218
   "resistance trance" 87
   utilizing 69, 84, **218f,** 220
Resources **281f**
Response
   abilities **178**
   attentiveness 67f, 80, 152
   delay 75
   readiness 152, 203
Reverse
   effect law 90
   set 55

suggestion 84f
Right-hemispheric functions 67f
   hypnosis and 201
   imaginative and 201
   symbolic and 201
   ultradian and 269
Robert 8, 124
Ryan, M. 267, 271

Scalp ulcers 170
Schizophrenia
   communication in 271
   hypnosis and 202
Secrets
   ideodynamics of 297
   inner life and **253f**
Segmentation phenomenon
   catalepsy as 82
   trance 204
Self-creation **299**
   dreams and **259f**
   posthypnotic 295
Sensory interassociations 66, 180
Sexual problems 125
Smoking 172
Somatic (processes)
   aiding 155
   interrelationships 166
Somnambulism 27, 30, 264
Speech
   problem reframed 293
   stuttering 296f
Stage hypnosis **178f**
Study improvement 122
Subject selection 43
Subjective experience
   time 195
   transforming 41, 158
Substitution 39

Suggestion (hypnotic) **17**
   all possibilities of response 178, 253
   as response-evoking ideas 20
   behavioral inevitabilities 144
   compound 60
   contingent 71, 85
   eye closure 92
   fail-safe 297
   for thumbsucking 20, 116
   ideas 20
   implication 21
   indirect 19, **283f**
   interspersed 298
   multilevel **275**
   multiple **213**
   naturalistic **16**
   open-ended 133, 297
   paradoxical 84, 116, 207, 235
   posthypnotic (*See separate listing*)
   progressive 166
   reverse 84, 116
   tactile 111, 155
   three-stage 75
   unconscious review 130
   utilizing lecture learnings 130
Summation 99, 103
Surprise
   casual 263
   "unexpected things" 273
Symptom
   analysis and **168**
   change **168, 207f**
   compulsive movement 207
   correction 167
   neurotic 259
   prescription 84, 116, **207**
   rechanneling 279
   reframing 169, 207, 279
   removal 118, 128, **299**

Symptom *(Cont'd)*
    signals 279
Synthetic (constructive)
    Method **251f**

Tactile *(See* Touch)
Techniques of suggestion 39
Therapeutic
    analogies **251f**, 255, **257f**,
        281, **291f**, 294
    dreams 259
    guides **276**
    metaphors **270**
    processes **270**
    work 253, **255f**, **275f**
Therapeutic hypnosis *(See also*
        Trance)
    defined **255f**
    essence of **235**
Thompson, Kay 234
Thumbsucking 20, 116
Tics 37
Time (temporal)
    considerations 151
    limitations as bind 190
    reorientation 195, 198, 199
    values 158, 160, 166
Time distortion
    cancer pain 24, 158
    facilitating **286f**
    mental climax and 285
    training 194
    trance indicator 75
Time double binds **10, 12,** 19
Touch (tactile)
    arm and hand levitation 87,
        154
    cues 87
    fixating attention 14
    suggestions for catalepsy 155
    suggestions for hand
        levitation 111

Trance
    active **266f**
    authoritative-participation
        approach 162
    awakening 92, 295
    building up 161
    catharsis in 119
    creative 269
    deepening 57f
    future 133
    goals 204
    ideomotor movement in 52
    indicators 112
    inducing 46, 67, 161, 210
    light 162
    physical contact in 111
    ratification 43, 78, 87, 112,
        235, **244f, 288f**
    readiness 72
    re-entering 23
    re-inducing (revivifying) 106,
        109, 133, 136, 139
    remembering vs.
        forgetting 126
    resistance 69
    "resistance trance" 87, 90
    segmentation 204
    self-discovery of 74
    somnambulistic 27, 30, 264
    successful 125, 150
    talking 217
    termination 82
    therapeutic 80
    via reverse set 55
    without awareness 38, 46,
        59, 145, 268
    work **266f**
Transcendant function **250f**
Transference **248f**
    indirect 256
Traumatic experience 21
    conscious mind and 120

Robert's truck accident 123
Trichotillomania 167
"Triple-layed recognition" 151
Truisms 19, 245, 255

Ultradian rhythms 52, 67, 246, 256, 268
Uncertainty 237
Unconscious (processes) 17, 119, **193**
  accessing 247
  aid 155, 172
  autonomous 247, 294
  choice 256
  cooperation 266, **287**
  corrective abilities 139
  creative **251f**
  directing ideas to 152
  direction 193
  dynamics 282
  feeling 256
  hypnosis and 225
  independent activity **144**
  knowledge 210
  learnings 46, 144, 263
  level 245
  listening with 143
  mind 50, **225f, 232f**
  nature **1f**
  potentials **257f**
  problem-solving 51, 282
  responding 240, 277f
  selection 51
  superior judgment of 117
  thinking 256
  trusting 53
  utilizing 52, **232f**
  work **272, 279f, 281f**
Understanding
  lack of 152
  reframing **10**

Urinary problems
  adult 192
  childhood 191
Utilization (utilizing) xiii, **1f**
  approaches 116
  associative network 245
  autohypnosis 64
  behavior **21**
  "climbing on board" 13
  confrontation 35
  control 184
  emotions 271
  experiential learning **225f, 228f, 232f**
  ideomotor head movements 43
  interests 248
  lecture learnings 130
  need for answers 148
  patient's viewpoint 170
  psychophysiological 105
  rational reasons 273
  reserve bank of life experiences 3
  resistances 69, 84, 220
  staring 261
  theory **257f,** 279
  trance 67
  unconscious 52
  wondering 261

Validity
  ideomotor cues 210
Vasectomy 198
Visualization (visual)
  approaches 214f
  hallucination 217
  hypnotic **214f**
Voice (vocal)
  dynamics 152
  fixation and 39
  tone reversals 235

Waking state
  catharsis in 119
"Wanting to want" **271**
Wilber, Ken xv
Wishing
  utilizing pain control 176
Wonder 141f, 148, 149, 167, **264**
  evoking 219, 262, 284
  inner search 257
Work **266f**
  active trance **266f, 270, 287f**

  evoking 281
  therapeutic **275f**
  unconscious **272f, 279f**
"Wounded Physician" xv

Yes set 19, 254, 275

Zen
  meditation and group 174